A Dynamic Materia Medica of the Noble Gases

ARGON

and elements of the third period

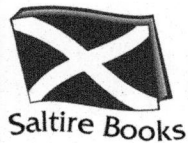

Saltire Books   *Saltire Books Limited, Glasgow, Scotland*

A Dynamic Materia Medica of the Noble Gases

ARGON

and elements of the third period

Jeremy Sherr

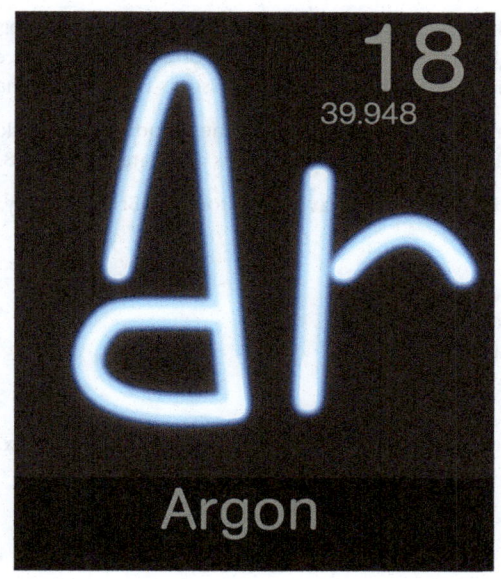

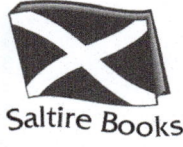

Saltire Books   *Saltire Books Limited, Glasgow, Scotland*

Published by Saltire Books Ltd

18–20 Main Street, Busby, Glasgow G76 8DU, Scotland
books@saltirebooks.com   www.saltirebooks.com

Cover, Design, Layout and Text © Saltire Books Ltd 2018

 is a registered trademark

First published in 2018

Typeset by Type Study, Scarborough, UK in 9¼ on 13½ Stone Serif
Printed and bound in the UK by TJ International Ltd, Padstow, Cornwall

ISBN 978-1-908127-30-3

For Saltire
Project Development: Lee Kayne
Editorial: Steven Kayne
Designer: Phil Barker
Indexee: Laurence Errington
Illustrator: Matt Canning
Additional graphics produced by Brenda Brown (brenda@brendapix.com)

CONTENTS

This book is dedicated to my fireball daughter,
Ella Naomi Sarah Sherr, may she find true love

... But this laborious, sometimes very laborious, search for and selection of the homoeopathic remedy most suitable in every respect to each morbid state, is an operation which, notwithstanding all the admirable books for facilitating it, still demands the study of the original sources themselves, and at the same time a great amount of circumspection and serious deliberation, which have their best reward in the consciousness of having faithfully discharged our duty. How could this laborious, care-demanding task, by which alone the best way of curing diseases is rendered possible, please the gentlemen of the new mongrel sect, who assume the honourable name of homoeopathists, and even seem to employ medicines in form and appearance homoeopathic, but determined upon by them anyhow (quid quid in buccam venit), and who, when the unsuitable remedy does not immediately give relief, in place of laying the blame on their unpardonable ignorance and laxity in performing the most important and serious of all human affairs, ascribe it to homoeopathy, which they accuse of great imperfection (if the truth be told, its imperfection consists in this, that the most suitable homoeopathic remedy for each morbid condition does not spontaneously fly into their mouths like roasted pigeons, without any trouble on their own part).

Samuel Hahnemann[1]

... the "accumulation" of electrons is continuous, so it would be more accurately depicted as a continuous spiral ribbon, a widening vortex rolling around itself like a seashell, cochlea, galaxy, and the musical scale. The eye, or center of gravity, of this spiral map of matter falls along the column of noble gases, because of their disdain for joining other elements in chemical bonding. They are the stable elements of the universe, balanced and complete unto themselves. .... A look at their atomic numbers shows the noble gases to have qualities of electrons very close to numbers from the Fibonacci sequence.

Symbol	Name	Atomic number	Closest Fibonacci Number
He	Helium (sun)	2	2
Ne	Neon (new)	10	8
Ar	Argon (inert)	18	21
Kr	Krypton (hidden)	36	34
Xe	Xenon (stranger)	54	55
Rn	Radon (ray)	86	89

MS Schneider[2]

References

1 Hahnemann S. Footnote to §149. *The Organon of the Healing Art* (6th edn). New Delhi: B Jain Publishers Pvt Ltd, 2003.
2 Schneider MS *A Beginner's Guide to Constructing the Universe*. New York NY: Harper, 1995. pp181–2.

ACKNOWLEDGEMENTS

A proving is a product of many people acting As If One Person, and so is this book. My thanks and gratitude go to the following friends and colleagues, without whom this book could not have manifested.

To the students of Dynamis Ireland 1996, who happily proved and sadly sang.

To David Retford for editing, nursing and holding this proving.

To Silvie Gowen for her extraordinary provings and her dedication in recording them. Silvie's amazing ability to hear the subtle universal currents has given all the Dynamis provings an extra dimension. Thank you Silvie!

To Dynamis Copenhagen for interrupting my lesson with a quick Argon proving. Ha-ha!

To Tina Quirk and Rebecca Stirrup for most excellent help with editing, advice, and inserting references, which I am incapable of doing. By always challenging me you have made this a better book by far!

To Naomi Jones, Cara Campbell and Rafi Neu for proof reading and advice.

To Anne Baker for re-editing the Argon proving.

To Brenda Brown, my wonderful illustrator, pictures speak better than words.

To John Morgan from Helios pharmacy for preparing the remedy and for supporting the noble art of proving.

To Yoram Verete, my teacher of Jewish studies.

To my publishers Steven and Lee Kayne of Saltire Books, for doing what all publishers should do, only better.

To Michal Yakir for expert botanical advice.

To all those who sent Argon cases: Charlotta Åström-Lynch, David Johnson, Sara Kabariti, Camilla Sherr and Kate Gathercole. Sujit Chatterjee for Banyan proving.

To my spiritual mentor Yaakov Melamed Cohen.

To my wife Camilla, for her love, support and inspiration, and for crying while reading my poems.

To all those that have supported me through the years, and for those I forgot to mention – Thank you!

All poems by J Sherr unless indicated otherwise.

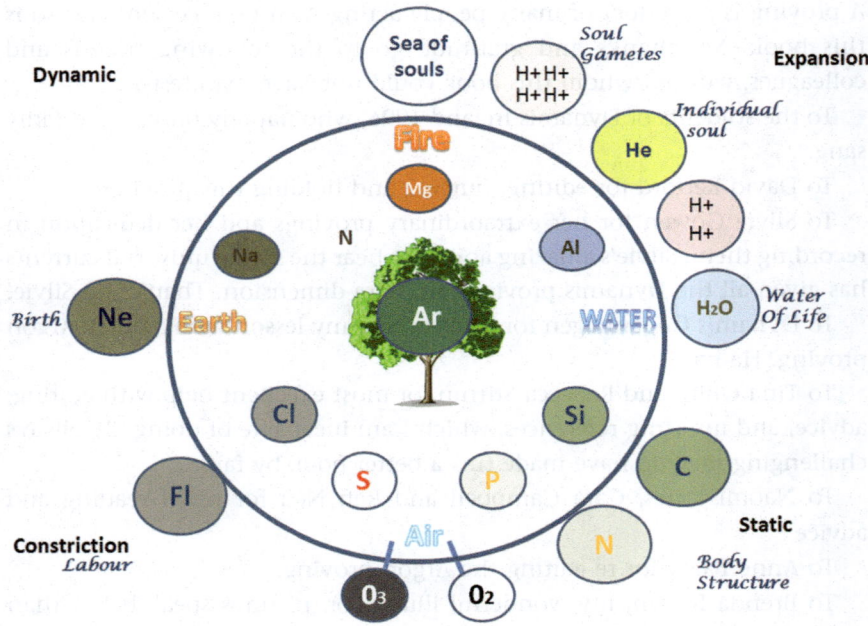

The Spiral Periodic Table (See Appendix for a full explanation)

ABOUT THE AUTHOR

Jeremy Sherr has practised homoeopathy for over 30 years. He practises in London, New York and Tel Aviv and is Principal of The Dynamis School for Advanced Homoeopathic Medicine that offers one of the oldest post graduate courses in the world today. Jeremy has taught homoeopathy throughout the USA and Europe as well as in Canada, China, India, Mexico, Japan, Russia, South Africa, New Zealand and Australia. He has conducted 34 classical homoeopathic provings and is the author of The Dynamics and Methodology of Homoeopathic Provings, Dynamic Provings Volumes I and II, Dynamic Materia Medica – Syphilis, Dynamic Materia Medica – Helium, Repertory of Mental Qualities and The Dynamic Case Taker. He has published numerous articles on homoeopathy and has conducted several research programmes. Since 2008, Jeremy has been living in Tanzania. Together with his wife Camilla, he has established several rural clinics and is working in the local hospital. They have treated over 6000 AIDs patients and have established food programmes and a day care centre for children with AIDs.

ILLUSTRATION CREDITS

Argon, number 18 by Brenda Brown (www.webtoon.com).
Spiral periodic table by Jeremy Sherr.

INTRODUCTION

The proving of Argon took place in Ireland with the Dynamis class of 1996. At the same time Dynamis UK undertook the proving of Krypton. The stark contrast between the two groups remains vivid in my memory. The Krypton group seemed depressed, heavy, even suicidal. At the same time the Argonites, as they later playfully called themselves, were cheerful, flowing and full of energy. Everyone seemed jubilant and light-hearted, as if a new dimension had opened up. However when the two groups met for a joint end-of-year party the polarities reversed. At our cabaret the Kryptonites got playful and rowdy while the Argonites melted into a weepy Nat-mur state, singing Irish love songs for those lost at sea. I was baffled. Perhaps it was an English-Irish divide.

I have since conducted several extra Argon provings with Dynamis Copenhagen, Silvie Gowen and my wife Camilla. Again the same picture emerged: a happy, cheerful energetic state – almost glowing. Due to the jubilant state, the Argon pathology was initially difficult to perceive. Not many patients complain of an easy, joyful and smooth life. Naturally, there is always another side. As in Neon, the challenge would be to perceive the 'negative'.

Writing this book has unfolded hidden facets of this remedy, and Argon has since become a frequent visitor to my clinic. Each symptom is a fractal of the whole, and the whole must be viewed in all its aspects. If we make do with two-dimensional emotional essences, our understanding will remain superficial. By studying the proving in detail, we can dive deeper, uncovering further dimensions from which much wisdom may be gained.

What is most striking is that all the Argon provings showed a remarkable consistency of meaning, a common denominator that ties the totality of symptoms together and dovetails perfectly into our noble gas journey.

We enter the magic garden of the third noble gas, Argon.

Jeremy Sherr
April 2018

1

THE POTENCIES OF PERCEPTION

In this book the levels of perception of the remedy equate with levels of potency. We can roughly compare the mother tincture level to the study of the element and its chemical properties, while the higher potencies of perception penetrate the innermost nature of the remedy's simple substance. This division into levels of potency is an analogy and has nothing whatsoever to do with the potencies taken by the provers. Nor are these potencies in any way related to the potency of prescriptions in clinical cases. The chapters Argon 12C or 30C do not relate to potency selection in prescribing, but to levels of perception. The potency should be selected according to the totality of the case regardless of which chapter the symptom lies in.

We can compare the study of argon, the element, to the basic mother tincture potency of perception, while the higher potencies of perception penetrate the innermost nature of the remedy's geometrical structure, metaphors and cosmic connotations.

Here is a summary of levels of potency equated with levels of perception, ranging from the gross to the subtle:

- *The element* represents purely chemical properties.
- *The mother tincture* represents homoeopathic preparation and naturopathic use, the realm of atoms and molecules.
- *The 12C level* represents physical affinities, the realm of organs.
- *The 30C level* represents general themes, the realm of the organism.
- *The 200C* represents essence, emotional pictures and signatures.
- *The 1M and 10M* potencies are an unravelling of the symptom configuration, a search for unified meaning in the totality.
- *The 50M* represents subtle sensations and functions, including the geometrical structure of the remedy picture.
- *The CM* explores the world of analogy and metaphor.
- *The MM* and beyond are an investigation into the esoteric roots of the remedy and the universal blueprint that lies beyond.

According to the 'grammatical' method of analysis, the 12C and 30C represent nouns, the 200C and 1M are adjectives and adverbs, while the 50M represents verbs, movement in time and space.[1] The potencies beyond transcend grammar to touch the language of poetry. Matching the remedy to the patient on the higher potencies of similarity will lead to deeper results, however for optimum similarity, all levels fit.

The notion of each potency level corresponding to a concept is not precise, but rather a general idea. The creation of yet another methodology to which homoeopaths should adhere can only lead to rigid prescribing.

Cases are included after the 50M section because most Argon cases can be solved from knowledge gained from the 12C to the 50M levels of perception. The higher-level chapters of CM and above relate to simple substance and thus to broader concepts than the individual remedy. Not everyone will feel comfortable with the information in these high-potency chapters. That is fine; there is no need to go there. I enjoy thinking of these things and maybe some readers will, too.

Only a few selected quotes from the provings have found their way into each section. Please be aware that it is important to read the proving as a whole to gain a thorough understanding of the remedy, as many symptoms only appear in the unabridged proving document.

Finally, when capitalised, Argon refers to the homoeopathic remedy, while argon in lower case refers to the basic element. All original symptoms from the Argon proving are given as follows: Argon symptom. Some proving symptoms have been abbreviated, or grammar has been corrected, without changing the essential content. The complete and original wording can be found in the full proving text itself. Keywords and phrases considered important are occasionally marked **in bold** within the proving.

Reference

1   Sherr J. *Dynamic Materia Medica – Syphilis: A Study of the Syphilitic Miasm* (2nd edn). Glasgow: Saltire Books, 2015.

ARGON THE ELEMENT

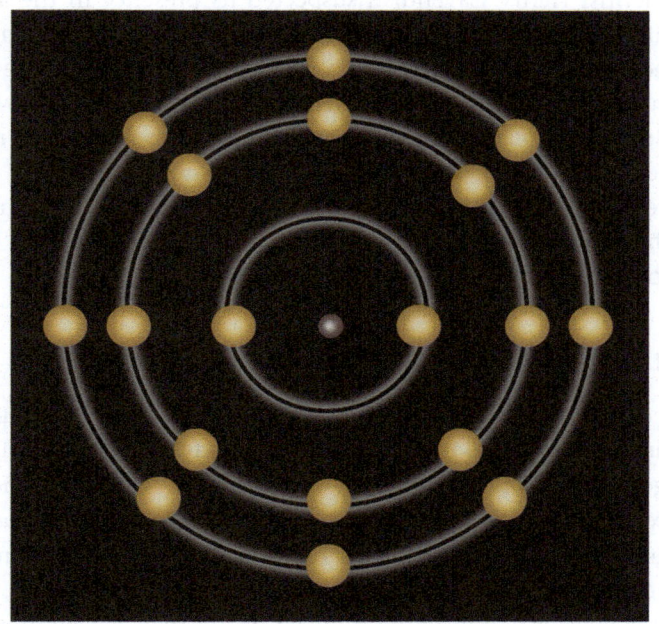

Figure 2.1 *Argon atom*

Element number 18, argon, is the third element of the noble gas series. It is colourless, odourless, tasteless and nontoxic in both its gaseous and liquid forms. The word argon comes from Greek meaning 'lazy' or 'idle' due to its chemical inactivity. The symbol for argon is Ar, however until 1957 it was simply known as A.

Argon is the third most common gas in the Earth's atmosphere, at 0.93%. Interestingly the Martian atmosphere contains approximately 2% argon by volume, Mercury's atmosphere contains 70% argon and radioactive argon-40 has been detected on Titan, Saturn's largest moon.

Argon's outer shells both have a complete set of eight electrons, which makes it very stable and resistant to molecular bonding. At room temperature argon does not form stable compounds, however it may combine with fluorine and hydrogen to create argon fluorohydride (HArF). Argon-containing ions, such as ArH^+ and ArF, are also known to exist.

History of discovery

Argon was the first member of the noble gases to be discovered. In 1775 British scientist Henry Cavendish suspected its presence in the air. It was not until 1894 however that Lord Rayleigh and Sir William Ramsay concluded that there was another gas mixed with nitrogen in the air. They had found that nitrogen produced from chemical compounds was half a percent lighter than nitrogen occurring in the atmosphere. By removing the oxygen, carbon dioxide, water and nitrogen from a sample of clean air, they were able to isolate argon. Several years before, H.F. Newall and W.N. Hartley had observed new lines in the colour spectrum of air, but were unable to identify the element responsible for the lines.

Production

As argon constitutes nearly one percent of the atmosphere by volume, most of the purified argon used in industry is produced from air. Argon is isolated by cryogenic fractional distillation, a process in which liquefied gases, argon, oxygen and nitrogen, are separated by heating them to their different boiling points. Liquid nitrogen boils at 77.4 K, while argon boils at 87.3 K, hence boiling at different temperatures can separate them. All other noble gases (except helium) are produced in this way as well, but argon is the most plentiful since it has the highest concentration in the atmosphere. Because argon is a by-product of the extraction of liquid oxygen and liquid nitrogen from the air, both of which are used on a large industrial scale, it is relatively inexpensive to produce. About 700,000 tons of argon are produced worldwide every year.

Applications

Lighting

Incandescent lights are filled with argon, to preserve the filaments from oxidation at high temperatures. Argon will not react with the filaments even in intense heat.

Argon is also used for the specific way it ionizes and emits light, such as in plasma globes. Gas-discharge lamps filled with argon provide blue light. Argon is used to create blue and green laser light.

Asphyxiant

Argon is considered highly dangerous in closed areas. In 1994 a man was asphyxiated after entering an argon-filled section of an oil pipe under construction in Alaska. Although argon is non-toxic, it depletes air of the normal level of oxygen, leading to suffocation. It is difficult to detect because it is colourless, odourless and tasteless.

Argon is used as an asphyxiant in the poultry industry, either for mass culling following disease outbreaks, or as a means of slaughter said to be more humane than the electric bath. Argon's relatively high density causes it to remain close to the ground during gassing. Its non-reactive nature makes it suitable in food production, and since it replaces oxygen within the dead bird, argon also enhances shelf life.

Because it reduces oxygen, argon is sometimes used for extinguishing fires where damage to equipment is to be avoided.

Preservative

Argon is often used as a preservative, in packaging material to displace oxygen and in moisture-containing air in order to extend the shelf life of products (argon has the European food additive code of E938). Museum conservators store important documents, such as the U.S. Declaration of Independence and Constitution, and the British Magna Carta, in argon-filled cases to retard their degradation.

Aerial oxidation, hydrolysis and other chemical reactions that destroy products, are retarded or prevented entirely by argon. High-purity chemicals and certain pharmaceutical products are sealed in bottles or ampoules packed in argon. In wine-making, argon is used to top-off barrels to avoid the aerial oxidation of ethanol to acetic acid during the aging process. In aerosol cans argon preserves compounds such as varnish, polyurethane, paint, etc. for storage after opening. In graphite electric furnaces, an argon atmosphere keeps graphite from oxidising.

Other applications of argon

- As an inert gas shield in many forms of welding, including metal inert gas welding and tungsten inert gas welding. For metal inert gas welding, argon is often mixed with CO_2.
- As the gas of choice (in ionised form) for sputter coating of specimens for scanning electron microscopy.
- As a protective atmosphere for growing silicon and germanium crystals and in partial-pressure heat treatment furnaces.
- As thermal insulation in energy efficient windows.
- In technical scuba diving to inflate a dry suit, because it is inert and has low thermal conductivity.
- As lasers in surgery to weld arteries, destroy tumours and to correct eye defects.
- In microelectronics for sputtering.
- For ice core and ground-water dating, since the half-life of argon-39 isotope is 269 years.

Medical uses of argon

- In the pharmaceutical industry to top off bottles of intravenous drug preparations (for example intravenous paracetamol), displacing oxygen and prolonging the drug's shelf life.
- In cryosurgery procedures, such as cryoablation, used as liquefied argon to destroy cancer cells.
- In surgery, used in 'argon enhanced coagulation', a form of argon plasma beam electrosurgery. The procedure carries a risk of producing gas embolism in the patient and has resulted in the death of one person via this type of accident.[1]

Reference

1   Palmer M, Miller CW, van Way CW 3rd, Onon EC. Venous gas embolism associated with argon-enhanced coagulation of liver. *J Invest Surg* 1993 Sep–Oct 6(5):391–9. Available online at: https://www.ncbi.nlm.nih.gov/pubmed/8292567

3

ARGON MOTHER TINCTURE

Argon was prepared and potentised at Helios Pharmacy in Tunbridge Wells, UK as follows:

Pure argon gas was sourced from BOC Pureshield® Argon. Product No. UN1006.

Argon was bubbled through purified water for 20 minutes to prepare a saturated solution at 20°C.

Solubility in water: 5 cc per 100 cc at 20°C.

This solution was regarded as 1C even though the amount dissolved was not determined.

This was diluted 1 in 100 in 50% alcohol to prepare the 2C. Higher potencies were made in 90% alcohol.

4

ARGON 12C PHYSICAL AFFINITIES

The main affinities of the Argon proving are respiration, asthma, chest, cough throat, stomach, head, eye, nose, digestion, kidney, bladder, skin, shoulder, coccyx and possibly sperm. For a complete list of physical symptoms refer to the full proving, available at www.dynamis.edu

So far, clinical cases have been helped in the mental-emotional spheres, with confirmed physical affinities of headaches, chest pain, itchy eczema, acne and warts.

5

ARGON 30C GENERALITIES

General symptoms that have emerged from the proving are:

- Alternating states switching between high energy and tiredness, followed by complete exhaustion.
- General dryness with the desire for bathing and walking in the rain.
- Extreme thirst, with a parched, dry feeling.
- Frequent and profuse urination.
- Urgent and sudden diarrhoea, which might be explosive.
- Fluctuations in appetite ranging from extreme hunger to aversion to eating.
- Desire for warm, comforting baby food, bread, chocolate, milk, onion and sweets, and aversion to sweets and tea.
- General aggravation from alcohol.
- Soreness and pain in breasts.
- Pain in chest and difficult respiration.
- Disturbed sleep with insomnia, waking and unrefreshed sleep.
- A sensation of heat occasionally described as glowing heat. Other provers experienced chills.

6

ARGON 200C EMOTIONAL ESSENCE

Argon shares some characteristics with the other nobles, such as the desire to be alone, tranquility, perfectionism and a need to be straight with the truth. Naturally it has its own unique character as well. Rather than the spiritual enlightenment of Helium or the contented bliss of Neon, the strongest impression of Argon is of playful happiness and ease. A cheerful and glowing state of mind is apparent. Argon people may be optimistic, bubbly and lighthearted, attracted to colour and harmony. Tasks seem easier to achieve, obstacles are removed and journeys flow with effortless ease, as if dancing or flying through life. Provers were industrious and full of energy, possessing a sense of clarity, synchronicity and connection with the universe. They appreciated the beauty of nature, sunsets, the earth and seas, the plants and the trees.

Argon displays many aspects of childhood ranging from infancy to teenage years. Provers had dreams of babies or sensations of being a baby, wanting to be breastfed, nurtured or wrapped in cosy, pink blankets. Patients may exhibit childish playfulness or the character of a naïve adolescent, using teenage language or falling into puppy love; perhaps like a young maiden waiting for her perfect young hero to ride in on a white horse. Hollywood abounds with examples of heroic and romantic 'coming of age' Argon movies, catering to nostalgia for a beautiful period of time most of us have experienced and lost. In reality, these romances often end with disillusionment, and Argon spans this side as well. If these romantic ideas do not work out, an intense state of grief may be experienced. The development, or non-development, of emotional maturity and the ability to integrate one's feelings and to form harmonious relationships are important aspects of Argon. This concept brings us to the negative side of the remedy.

Argon may remain in the innocent state of a child and be unable to accept adult roles and responsibility. Protection is an important theme – the child-like Argon needs security, and will suffer if they feel unprotected. Patients can be anxious, depressed, tearful, indolent, irritable, restless, sad and even deceitful. The positive and negative states can alternate sharply. Like the other noble gases, Argon can be wrapped in self-obsession and find it difficult to see and truly interact with those around, thus making for an interesting but ultimately dry personality.

In the proving there was an impression of chaotic disorder and unsuccessful efforts to achieve things, a sensation that the free flow of life was impeded by accidents, blocked roads and missed appointments, flights and opportunities. Hence Argon may have a dislike of deadlines, restrictions or obstructions. Provers were forgetful, made mistakes, wasted time and postponed tasks, resulting in a guilty feeling or a desire to escape from the confines of civilisation. Naturally there was a degree of irritability, sometimes manifesting as assertive behaviour, 'remove the obstacles and let me through'.

I vividly remember an unpleasant incident that I had during the proving. As is often the case I did not realise the connection at the time, and it was only once I understood the remedy that it became clear to me that this had been part of my Argon proving. I was in Ireland teaching Dynamis, and a good friend of mine came to visit. I decided to take his family and mine on a trip to Dingle on the west coast so that we could see the beautiful views and sea, perhaps even a dolphin playing. The trip turned out to be a nightmare I will never forget. The car was slow and had no power. I drove much more carefully than usual because I was anxious about the mothers and babies in the back. The trip was full of delays, the roads were narrow and we were stuck behind slow vehicles for hours, unable to overtake. Nothing flowed. The supposedly two-hour journey lasted eight hours. We arrived in the dark, tired and irritable, and spent two more hours looking for a hotel. No one had a good time, my friends were angry and I was so frustrated that I burst into tears.

During my time teaching the Argon group, I managed to miss six flights to Ireland, either due to my own fault or airline chaos. While I am often a last-minute person, I had never missed a flight before. (These symptoms may also be part of Krypton, I had been proving both consecutively).

Argon may have dreams or images of being buried in the earth. Other miscellaneous phenomena were the tendency to lose and to find things. Provers had images and dreams of crocodiles, otters, fairies, mermaids, cats, fish, jade and rose quartz.

One strange phenomenon was that a number of people reported many light bulbs blowing in their houses. Of course, this is related to the industrial use of argon in light bulbs. I have since confirmed this 'symptom' in practice.

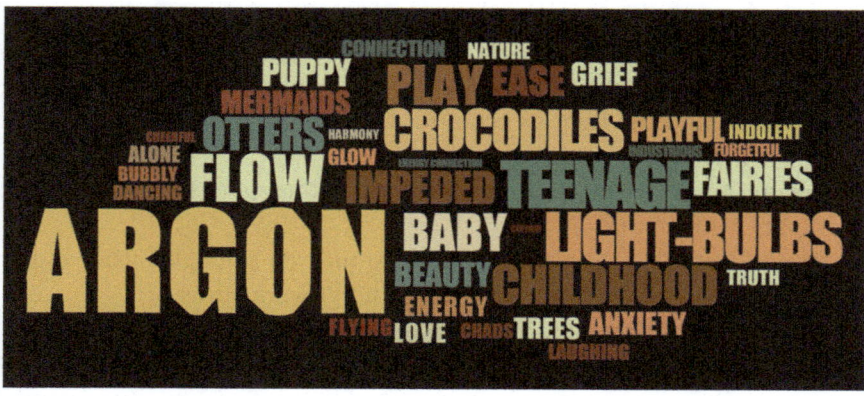

Figure 6.1 Argon wordle

Lights and Electricity Blowing

Sensation – I am enclosed in a light bulb.

I am very aware of the huge number of light bulbs that have blown over the past three weeks. Never in 20 years have I had to replace that number: 17 bulbs in one month!

Altogether during the proving I replaced 6 bulbs.

Light bulbs kept blowing in the house. We seemed to be buying and replacing light bulbs much more often than usual.

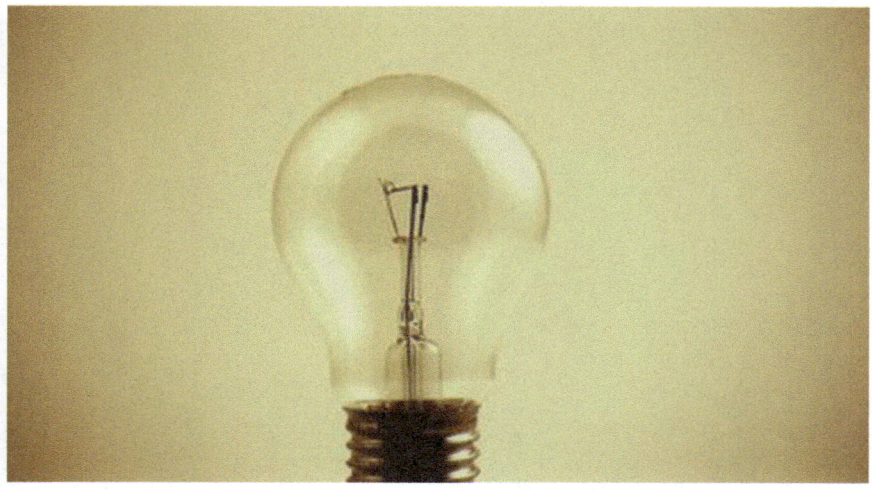

Figure 6.2 Electric light bulb

Three light bulbs blown today.

Dream in a large flat, in an old building with a group of people, we had just moved in, the lighting was bad. Went around trying various switches, eventually found the right switches for the lights. I was disturbed by lack of lighting, panicky.

Dream: An old friend from childhood was there and kept turning out the lights, which annoyed me.

Dream: Getting out of bed and tried to turn on the lights, they didn't work, went into my mother's, her lights didn't work either.

The kettle short-circuited and the toaster blew.

I was glowing and others thought so too!

7

ARGON 1M
HIGHER EMOTIONAL THEMES

Roll up for the magical mystery tour through Argon-land!

Our journey begins with the characteristic contentment, calmness and tranquility shared by many of the noble gases. It then flows into the euphoric state peculiar to Argon, a state glowing with happiness, good energy and an ease of being. From there we will effortlessly grow into infancy, tightly wrapped in our mother's pink, snuggly blankets. We will then graduate into the light-speckled gardens of childhood, charmed with magical beings, fairies, playful otters, butterflies, crocodiles and pirates. Into this magical land of limitless possibilities, we fly, we will never grow up! No duties here to constrict our life, no ticking clocks or adults to shadow our light. But when childhood buds blossom into flowers and hormones flow, our attention will turn from the birds and bees to the wafting scents of love and sex, tumbling into the perfect romance that will, 'like OMG, soooo last forever'.

There is no need to elaborate on each of the themes that appears in this section, as the proving symptoms speak clearly for themselves.

Alone

As if I am totally alone.

Calm

Glass jar leapt from fridge. I reacted calmly despite the greasy chaos it caused.

After the car accident I was dead calm, despite my normal reaction to even the sound of a distant car crash, when I would be shaking and choking back tears.

Since the proving I have the sense that any loss or accident or oversight is okay because nothing fatal can happen and everything comes right.

Content

Contented smiley feeling, like a cat that licked the cream.

Feeling of clarity of thought and of deep connection. Energy very high and focused. Complete feeling of change within body. Feeling of flowing. Feeling alive and feminine. Feeling of serenity.

A feeling of completion, don't need food or anything else.

I feel a kind of soft wholeness and roundness, light, happy and somehow content with myself, a nice feeling.

Inaction

Did not feel like working, happy to be and not to act.

Beauty

Nature, experience, everything was covered with frost flowers, soooo beautiful. A feeling of being soooo alive in this world.

Heightened appreciation of colours and beauty. Magic swim in pool by mountain shrouded in mists, glorious with autumn colours.

Standing on the balcony, I see all in super detail, all the colours are clear, sharp, nature is alive, sharp, detailed. I feel above it all, looking down on the wonderful world. Feel as if I could fly.

Laughter and fun

Got up to a strong smell of gas in the kitchen. Chatting with my son who gave me a lecture on not lighting matches or using anything electrical. I cannot stop laughing. He tells me it isn't funny at all.

Someone told me a funny joke and I almost went hysterical with laughing.

Laughing and joking with daughters – very unusual for this hour of the morning.

Infectious laughter.

Felt totally optimistic and bubbly.

I feel cheerful;

While thinking of this I am having a lot of fun.

I want to be funny! Must chat with friends more often;

We are gone, light headed, giggling, silly in whole class, happy, light, laughing silly.

Energy

Ease and contentment, energy level high.

Energy is better than normal. I feel really good on this remedy.

A great sense of energy, a surge of energy to complete tasks and objectives. A sense of having a great deal of power behind me, a huge support. Something was pushing me forward and there was no going back.

Glowing

People kept remarking that I was glowing, that I had a very glowing energy about me. A film crew came to the house to interview me for T.V. The director came into the house and she looked at me and said that I was glowing, a real healthy glow. The camera man commented about the glow all over the house. He filmed in three rooms in the house so he could catch the glow. On T.V. this glow was really evident.

Golden glowing light on left periphery during consultation yesterday – powerful. It happened again during the college weekend and last week in college – That makes 3.

Happiness

Happy walking in the rain, more noticeably happy.

Good happy feelings. I'm on top of things.

I have a feeling as if I am walking on clouds, euphoria.

Contented smiley feeling, like a cat who licked the cream.

Want to go back to my grandparent's home. I feel great love and connectedness with grandparents. Felt like crying with happiness.

Baby

Dream of an 18-month-old baby.

Desired to be wrapped up warm and safe.

Woke with a sense of peace and comfort as if cushioned in the softest warmest cloud.

Feel nurtured, like a child who has been breastfed and is lying in mother's arm, nestling, cosy, warm. All is well with the world.

Wanted to be wrapped in a soft blanket and held close like a baby crying with pure joy. Felt completely connected to my husband when he held me. Wanted to make love with him. Put a pink blanket on the bed and we wrapped up in it. I felt pure contentment and pure connectedness. My body is loose and free – everything is bright and warm. I want to stay with this feeling.

I had a bath. I felt I was a new-born baby having my first bath. I found a pink towel and baby powder that belonged to my mother. I felt she had left it there for me. I had a feeling of complete connectedness and I wanted to give this feeling to everyone. Ate muesli and milk – heated it – not too hot, not too cold – baby food. Longing for baby food.

I feel a kind of soft wholeness and roundness, light, happy and somehow content with myself, a nice feeling. I become curious, more and more and I took another dose.

Thought about breast milk, animals feeding their young.

I went to a photographer who has lost the old negatives of my son, before he grew up, which I wanted to reprint very badly.

Dreams about babies.

Dreamt my mother (81 years old) had a baby.

Dream I was much younger and had a job baby-sitting.

Went into my house and found 2 babies asleep in prams who I thought no one was minding. I went around, rushing, trying to make up bottles before the mothers came to collect them, thinking that had been neglected by whoever was supposed to be minding them. Later found my niece had been minding them all the time.

Innocent child-like

Great exhilaration and a desire to have fun.

I feel giggly, as if I'm high, like a child enjoying herself.

Playing in the water, walking with my arms – like being a little girl – memories of being a child.

Anxiety of not hearing children, or not being around to protect them.

Playful

Cheerful and benign today because I was out – freedom – lunch and Christmas shopping in gorgeous places. A day in the woods, so to speak, just playing.

Very playful tonight with my son.

Want to play and do fun things, go shopping.

Feel like going out, walk or cinema or something enjoyable.

Huge change at home. All 4 killer dogs behaving lovingly together. This wasn't ever possible since the pups grew up. This is extremely significant. My dogs have been the biggest test of this proving. The female is happy and playful. She used to keep out of the way. The dogs just express what we feel.

Dancing and singing

Bought *Dances with Wolves*.[i] Can't wait to watch the dance bit again.

It is a feeling as if I am dancing with a shadow.

It is like dancing in Tai Chi!

My dancing partner, a very good and experienced dancer, asked 'What has happened to you?' and I suddenly knew what she meant – the dancing was different. I felt softer roundedness in my movements. I was smiling all the time, my dance movements were softer, not making the old mistakes.

I felt like singing and dancing around the place – I couldn't stop smiling.

Teenager

My main feeling in the proving was of adolescence, perennial adolescence.

Dream I am in my late teens.

The word 'blithe' came up, meaning carefree and heedless of consequences. Irresponsible and carefree. When I look at myself being censorious, I think: 'You horrible, old farty person!'

---

[i] 1990 Oscar winning epic Western film (MGM).

Peter Pan

Desire to go to the balcony and jump out – nothing would happen and I would easily land on my feet.

Feel as if I could fly.

Dreams of flying.

It is a feeling as if I am dancing with a shadow.

The crocodiles' habitat is threatened by the destruction of trees. Is it a fairy tale, or a fairy tail, which is being told?

Delusion that I was a mermaid.

Dream I was making homes out of cardboard boxes and carpets, for lost boys.

Fairies

Dream of the word 'fairy'.

I feel like the fairies in that book where the girl catches them in her diary by snapping it shut suddenly and squashes them between the pages like a flower press.

Dream I had a little friend with short hair sticking up every way and coloured pink, green, and orange. She was like a fairy or a sprite. I thought she was wonderful, in contrast to my waking attitude to this adolescent hair and hyperactive mischief.

Puppy love

I found a picture of a very attractive man from Facebook, and I feel enchantment looking at him. Maybe I have always secretly liked his type of man, but I haven't noticed it before. He is blond and his chin and lips are strong. And he sounds really funny and intelligent. I feel I want this kind of man, but I can't be bothered to do anything to get him.

Singing while driving *Baby Love*[i] with accurate voice and style.

Dream I was being very beautiful, tried to attract a man in the store.

No duty

Anxiety about something I had not done to protect others. Responsibility; are we responsible for another when we are 18, are we responsible at 18?

---

[i] 1964 Song first recorded by American group The Supremes (Motown).

I suddenly noticed that I don't have a conscience.

Don't have structure, am just going around without being able to take any responsibility.

Creativity

I feel very positive, strongly focused, able to clear work that has been outstanding for months, very productive.

Very industrious all day.

Getting a lot of work done on house we intended to renovate for the last few years – painting, sanding and varnishing.

Generally more industrious, getting more jobs finished and finishing jobs which had been put off.

Extremely productive day – closed the practice.

Magic Garden

In the magic garden of my childhood
time frolicked and lingered,
never a factor.
I would like to tell of flowers,
of magic moments, of carefree laughter, but
It was not all glory
or fairies, no.
Little fears flashed behind trees,
sexual notions like butterflies
floating near,
admonitions of the old
lying heavy on my bed by night.
A mother, swallowed by the unexplained.
Confusion.
Who and what and why
But no what if's.
Still, it was my garden
and my thoughts were
free to wander unobstructed,
Rivulets of rain rolling winter windows
forming
purposeless puddles for long afternoons.
Perhaps a friend,
or dreaded school day.
Perfect? That cursed notion had not yet seized my being.
The freedom
was from
my own mind.

Negative side

In the previous section we examined the charmed and childish life of Argon. This behaviour would be the norm for age-appropriate patients. One would not prescribe Argon for a four-year-old acting immaturely, or a teenager falling in love for the first time. The challenge is to perceive this naïve, childish or teenage behaviour in an adult. It would be even more difficult to perceive this as an exaggerated tendency in a child.

Never-never land cannot last forever. If it does it will come at a price, the interest rate that time extracts. The ending of childhood highlights the other side of Argon, a depressed, isolated, irritable, angry, indolent and discontented condition, often stemming from a disillusioned state that cannot reconcile the burden of adulthood with the perfect and untainted world of a child. At worst this deteriorates into a chaotic loss of control, feeling trapped by circumstances that we are not capable of dealing with. The state may manifest in panic attacks and sharp changes of moods, perhaps a manic-depressive condition or feelings of persecution.

Our innocent trust, wrapped in baby blankets and nurtured by fairy tales, has been shattered. We are no longer the centre of mummy's universe. Our childhood has given way to a hard and aggressive world; we are over-whelmed by toil, trouble and a responsibility that is often symbolized by authority figures such as police or wardens. We can no longer get away with the things we used to. Sometimes, the only way we can deal with this deceitful world is by spinning our own web of deceit, a far cry from the truthful nobility of our adolescent ideals.

Disconnected

After that there was no connection between what was happening on the teacher's board and in my head. I could see what was happening, but it did not get into my head, a disconnection.

I felt very apart from everyone else – this was just my trip, nobody else was involved.

Exhaustion

Feeling very fatigued. Cannot concentrate.
Depressed. Feeling exhausted, unable to concentrate.
No desire to get out of bed.

Don't want to work.
Physically and otherwise exhausted.

Depressed

Feeling of deadness, nothingness, no soul, no spirit. Wanted to cry with disappointment, that I had **lost the feeling of completeness and connectedness**. There is a big empty void inside me. I am a walking corpse.
Feeling moody and sorry for myself.
Depressed. As if I am inadequate to perform my duties. Feel like weeping, but tears do not come.
Feeling depressed all day. Didn't want to communicate with anyone. Energy low – dragging myself around. Feeling unhappy and weepy.
Woke with a feeling of bleakness, a sense of hopelessness and lack of direction in my life.
Noticeably depressed and unsure about the future.

Grief

In the following symptoms note that alongside the grief is disillusionment at the loss of youth and childhood and an attempt to **preserve the past** by means of a plastic bag. All this is highly reminiscent of Natrum muriaticum, as we will later see.

Feels like no corrosion. I did not corrode, I was not responsible.
Dreamt of feeling sadness when neighbour talked about my mother who had died.
I started thinking about the 21-year-old boy that was killed working on the sewage between my house and my old house. As I sat here, it seemed horribly sad. I haven't been able to get it out of my mind all week. Tears have just welled up and I've been crying my eyes out. This was totally out of character for me. I don't even know who he was. It doesn't matter. This kid being buried alive is like a **monstrous disillusionment for a much younger self than my experienced, old soul**. Weeping overwhelms me at the thought of the **beautiful illusion, gone with this boy**.
Dream that my husband died. **We put him in a plastic bag** and tied it at the bottom so that he was completely sealed in the bag. We put him on a bed in a room. The next morning I found my small daughter fast asleep on top of him. The plastic bag was stuck to his face. [This was a terrible

image, the grief I felt for days later was dreadful. Even though I was aware that it was only a dream and my husband was alive and well, I just could not be consoled. The grief was awful.]

Driving and scanning the music channel. Get a pipe lament and realise I have tuned into the Remembrance Day programme from England, I remember an uncle killed in the war and connect with my grandmother's anguish – it expands to the anguish of all mothers – a profound sadness engulfs me. Elgar's music started and when the announcer began reciting a poem tears flowed down my cheeks. I prayed fervently for world peace. Arrived at my destination at exactly 11.00 as one-minute silence begins. A very strange feeling.

Felt sad it is the end of an era we are at now. Religion isn't here for a large degree of people and there's nothing else yet for the majority as a replacement. **Nostalgic for the past, an era is coming to the end** with my parent's generation.

Irritability

Not speaking with anyone at home. Feel as if I shall explode if anyone crosses me.

Extremely irritated with husband. Had a violent argument, which erupted quickly. He approached me in a threatening manner and I said to myself, 'if he comes one step closer I'll hit him with something.' I felt ready for a fight to the death, I was trembling and shouting with rage.

Unable to sleep due to husband's snoring. Woken four times. Becoming increasingly irritable. I yank the clothes from him and complain that he kept me awake all night. Seething with anger.

Feeling very irritable. Ameliorated by a long walk in the fresh air.

My husband found me very irritable, picking on him over silly things. I felt fine, felt I had a right to do it.

Very irritable and horrid to the checkout girl in supermarket, much worse than my usual. My daughter said I was very whingy in town too.

Very irritable and crabby today. Found myself muttering out loud on the street – to my dismay.

Three women were sitting surrounded by litter at end of weekend. When I asked them to help they ignored me. I urged them cheerfully and one said 'That's your issue'. I would expect this from New York, but not Ireland. I would usually bristle all over. I was just surprised.

In the bank noticed wrong coins in the wrong stack, felt irritated by it.

Feeling irritable with customers and colleagues, felt they were asking unnecessary questions, it annoyed me.

Extremely irritable. Shouting at the children and inclined to smack (unusual for me). My daughter got the first smack of her life. She was shocked. Also, very irritable with my husband. I totally over-react to his actions, shouting abuse at him.

Anger

I was really angry I couldn't get my supervisor all day.

Argued with husband over breakfast. Felt angry and stubborn.

Husband started to get sarcastic during a normal conversation. I suddenly became very angry. Mimicked back to him the way he was speaking, got up and left the table in a huff.

Woken by argument between husband and son. I became very angry and felt like physically assaulting my husband, I am aware of an inner explosive anger, which could erupt at the slightest provocation.

Short-lived anger with daughter over missed appointment. Unusual for me to respond like that.

Anger with business partner.

Felt very angry about racism story on radio.

Cannot understand why people have to fight. Like when someone says rude things to others, I feel sad and try to shut the energy out. Like when people say 'Idiot' or 'F**K you!'

(Inability to accept rude, adult behaviour – JS)

Panic attacks

Extraordinary sensation in my solar plexus, like an inner trembling, I feel anxious and my breathing is very restricted like a band around my chest, breathing shallow. I feel very jittery, nervous and nauseated, too nervous to drive.

A sensation of inner trembling. I felt it was going on and on and I couldn't stop it. I had no co-ordination, poor control, I lost cohesion and things seemed out of sequence. The sensation was confusion and a jittery feeling in the solar plexus. I was short of breath and like I'm panting short shallow breathing. The whole sensation lasted an hour accompanied by a feeling of anxiety.

Terrible racing heart before speaking in class.

It's all too much!

The following symptoms show the difficulty of living in an adult world and struggling to deal with children's chaos.

I live in a fish bowl in order to be near to my four telephones. My answer-phone makes my home into a crisis centre where 'time off' is never possible. Yesterday was a nightmare. I have no escape. I think a lot about drifting off to the other end of the earth somewhere – getting away from civilis-ation.

Disturbed by the dark forces of disorder and unable to restrain my temper with my teenage son's ineptitude and laziness. Besieged by emer-gencies and urgent tasks. Further behind than ever and mess everywhere. The accumulated junk of three years is dumped in the centre of the house instead of cleared away as planned. Chaos, which I'm supposed to fix quick. I don't know how to be a father. I don't have time to be a mother and still there is no space or time for my work. I feel alone and apprehensive, worse because of the dark morning. How can I create light and beauty and harmony when I am overpowered by disruption, horror films, junk food and accumulating trash?

Deeply disturbed, unable to sleep. Dogs barking, but the turbulence is in my head. Everything seems worse than it is. The leaking roof after the momentous rains isn't catastrophic but it feels like it. Abnormality seems to me like a fungus – people and roof beams, rotten underneath – I don't seem to have any safe place or safe time away from these things. The disorder in my perceived world is starting to breed and multiply out of control and there is never time to get to the source to stop the spread.

Deceitful

Unable to get my son out of bed. Told him a lie – that his drive was waiting for him at the gate.

Gave money to my son to go to the pictures. His grandmother criticises me allowing him out late at night. I defend him saying, 'he always goes to the pictures on Friday' while actually he doesn't.

(Defending the freedom of childhood, lying to her mother, like a child – JS)

Search my husband's wallet for money. Realise I am being deceitful. I have enough of my own. No remorse.

Felt the most effective way to terrorise someone was to tell lies.

Sensation that I was lying waiting, like I was horizontal lying but not telling lies lying.

I was saying the opposite sound or word to what I meant. It felt like there was disconnection between the mind and the mouth.

Aware that the truth is straight, deceit is crooked.

Police/theft/prison

The following symptoms portray the constriction from and mistrust of authority, of the forbidding adult world. A policeman is chasing an abandoned child, a man seeks attention and love but receives strict indifference, people are caught and imprisoned.

Dream In which the theme was not being able to trust people in society that one should be able to trust, e.g. the police.

Dream I was chasing a man, I was a Garda (police), chased him up an alley way, turned out he **was a child I had given up for adoption**. (Childhood lost – JS)

Dream a man pulled out a large scissors and stabbed a **policewoman** in the back, she just turned around and looked at him, **no expression**. I knew the reason he had done this was to bring **attention to himself**. (Mummy doesn't care anymore – JS)

Dreamt of shoplifting – stole an onion. Got caught and was brought to court. Things became twisted and exaggerated. Felt very scared. (Adult world, can't get away with things anymore – JS)

Dream of the house being broken into; felt the presence of someone in the house.

Dream of a prison camp – the women reduced to eating cosmetics from little plastic trays **like kid's paint boxes** and men and women are building and taking down fences made of barbed wire. (Child in the constraints of an adult world – JS)

Dream, I was in some kind of camp, I was like a warden.

8

ARGON 10M SPIRITUAL THEMES

Day Three

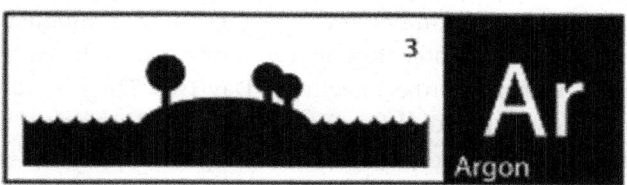

Figure 8.1 Argon Day Three

The main thing in my proving was the number three. Threes kept coming up all through the proving, over and over and over again.

Dream of spinning triangles and the number three.

In the previous two volumes of this series we examined the correspondence between the first two days of creation and Helium and Neon. It is pertinent to look for a similar correspondence in the proving of Argon and compare it with the third day of creation, and, indeed, the similarities are striking. What is important is not to just highlight these comparisons but to extract the meaning that arises from them towards a deeper understanding of Argon, its relationship to the third period and the relevant Biblical passage.

> And God said: 'Let the waters under the heaven be gathered together unto one place, and let the dry land appear.' And it was so. And God called the dry land Earth, and the gathering together of the waters He called Seas; and God saw that it was good.
>
> And God said: 'Let the earth put forth grass, herb yielding seed, and fruit-tree bearing fruit after its kind, wherein is the seed thereof, upon the earth.' And it was so. And the earth brought forth grass, herb yielding seed after its kind, and tree bearing fruit, wherein is the seed thereof, after its kind; and God saw that it was good. And there was evening and there was morning, a third day.[1]

Delusion the day started in the evening.

> Because on that day [second day – JS] divisiveness was created; as it is written, 'it
> shall divide between water and water.' However, the Midrash then goes on to
> point out that on the third day the phrase 'it was good' appears twice, because
> then 'the work of the waters,' which begun on the second day, was completed.[2]

As explained in the Neon book, the second day of creation is unique among
the days of creation, because it does not conclude with the phrase '. . . *and
God saw that it was good*'. This phrase, a symbol of completeness and
completion, represents the noble gas at the end of a period. Day Three, on
the other hand, is composed of two parts, each finishing with the words
'*And it was good*', representing two noble gases – Neon and Argon. It appears
that the unravelling of the second period and Neon is not completed at the
end of the second day as one might expect, but in the middle of the third
day. God withdraws the waters to one place and exposes the earth, completing the unfinished water project begun on Day Two. The second period and
Neon terminate at the end of the first part of Day Three with water-earth
separation and the noble exclamation '*It was good*'.

In the Neon proving we see the first appearance of land, as in the
symptom '*At last I touch the earth*'. This landing on earth is also well represented in the Neon clinical cases. While most of the remedy Neon seems
incredibly watery, this *dry land* represents the complementary opposite. In
both the Neon remedy picture and in the biblical story, earth appears, and
for the first time we have all four elements necessary for life: Fire, Air, Water,
Earth (hydrogen, oxygen, H_2O and the third period). Earth, as in the second
part of the biblical Day Three, is now fertile, and begins to produce
vegetation in the form of grass, plants, trees, fruit and seed, first life. By
producing seed this vegetation is able to reproduce and provide us with the
green, lush, varied, edible, beautiful and vital planet on which we live.

As the third period unfolds, the earthly elements are exposed and supply
the necessary ingredients for plant life. Natrum and chlorum, situated at
either end of the period, crystallise salt, which forms both the boundary
and the interplay of earth and sea. Alumina, from which clay and pots are
made, is the great separator of earth and water. Magnesium, alumina, silica,
sulphur and phosphorus are all essential ingredients of plant life. Thus, the
third period depicts both the exposure of earth and its vegetable offshoots.
Finally, combining all these elements in perfect completion, trees grow,
manifesting the perfect fertility of earth. Argon. *And it was good.*

Neon, which relates to water, is feminine in essence and its proving
portrays ova passively waiting for seeds to fertilize them. The ova flash their
alluring neon lights at passing knights. These knights, and the seeds they

carry, are not yet present in Neon, hence the ova cannot be impregnated to create fruit-bearing pregnancies. But on the third day, now that the relatively yang earth has become exposed, foreplay can begin, frolicking through childhood and working up to conception through a ripening adolescence whence seeds can be sown, conceive and sprout life. Labour and its consequent child-bearing responsibilities will not appear until the more demanding fourth period. Why think of these things when the summer fruit of love is so sweet?

The third day unfolds

As we will see in the following section, the developments of the third day can be tracked through the proving of Argon- from the earth's separation from water, to the rising of land, the growth of vegetation and seed and the garden of childhood. Let us take a walk through Argon and the creation of life on earth.

We begin with the gathering of water to expose the earth. At last we have something solid to stand upright on, to store our possessions and memories in, to claim as our territory, to be buried in.

Earth separates from water

Before the raven there was one big ocean, before land. After the raven magic there were rivers and springs and lakes and land. At that time the raven was silver white, not black.

This proving expression reminds us of a parallel biblical story, Noah and the flood. Noah was a noble, righteous and pure man who walked the straight path (Helium), until the flood occurred and the animals were 'arked' two by two for exactly ten months (Neon, period two, element number ten), and finally earth was exposed so plants and people could once again grow (Argon).

From the book of Genesis:

> And the waters decreased continually until the tenth month; in the tenth month, on the first day of the month, were the tops of the mountains seen. And it came to pass at the end of forty days, that Noah opened the window of the ark which he had made. And he sent forth a raven, and it went forth to and fro, until the waters were dried up from off the earth.[3]

Earth

As the waters separate, earth appears.

Dream the ground seemed to have crumbled away.

Felt a grounding, my legs connected to the ground.

A dream about being on a worn road, a lane, like the one we live on. It was strange how badly worn it was, like it was gone back into the earth.

I had an image of a corpse in a bog, being **preserved** for thousands of years. The following day I was coughing and the image was that I was coughing up dirt from being **buried alive**.

It felt like I was an animal burrowing into the earth with my hands.

Felt like the front of me was warm from the earth and back warm from the sun. This felt like total nourishment.

I started thinking about the 21-year-old boy that was killed working on the sewage between my house and my old house. A wall fell on him.

Dreamed about a monster – mythical, like the Loch Ness monster, which was to emerge from beneath the earth. No one would believe me. Then there were reports that its head had been sighted. I could see a crack along a huge land mass where the monster would emerge.

I heard noisy teenagers outside and became frightened. Got out of bed and tried to turn on the lights, they didn't work, went into my mother's, her lights didn't work either. Looked out a window, it was like dawn, saw a female neighbour shoving earth from a truck into another garden and thought that was the reason the **lights wouldn't come on**.

Earth and water

Now that we have both earth and water, they begin to form a relationship. Seas surround the earth, the tides rise and fall, puddles and swamps form.

There were fireballs and meteorites, but you're safe in water.

I live in a fish bowl . . . a refugee from a distant swamp.

Desire to go somewhere near the sea.

Dream I was a child given a book of tides.

Feel like I'm sliding backwards into murky waters.

Playing golf beside the sea. There was a high tide following the moon. I was acutely aware of the power and energy of the sea. Feeling exhilarated by the energy.

A little Belgian child told me after returning to Ireland from a summer spent in the lakes: 'My natural habitat is water!' I thought – Mine too!

Feeling of ease and contentment – connected to the Universe, the Earth, the Sea. Energy level high.

Dream of being urged to go into an outdoor swimming pool with contact lenses on – **I am in my late teens.**

Enjoyed contrast between smooth and knobbly. Protection is smooth.

(The contrast between rough earth and smooth water, or old and young – JS)

We moved outside to the sea front and were walking and dancing along.

Felt connected to earth and spirit. Sense of oneness, as if I would dissolve into energy of waves, sea, sand, sky.

People tell us we cannot bathe at that part of the beach. I just laughed at them, you cannot possess the sea.

Desire to go somewhere near the sea.

Dream of swimming by the beach, the water was stormy but suddenly changed to a clear calm tropical sea, warm and beautiful. The water was like heaven.

Felt very pleased with rubber, like it was the biggest gift that could be given. Even better than cork, because cork gets wet whereas rubber protects from the wet.

Earth and water are attracted to each other, but as yet there is no real intercourse between the two. Rubber separates the interaction of earth and water, as it does with male and female. The love-making between earth and water depends on the distillation of pure water from salty seawater through evaporation and the formation of clouds, rain and rivers. Only then can the Tree of Life grow. The water cycle is the most important aspect to develop in the third day. Without it there would be no vegetation or life on earth. This development requires an interaction between sun and water, cloud and cold front, rain and earth.

Watched the dawn break, it was really beautiful. When the **sun rose**, the sky was clear and bright orange, it looked magnificent with white **clouds** – no formation to them. **Sexual feelings.**

As if I am **walking on clouds**, euphoria.

Happy walking in the **rain**, more noticeably happy.

During the proving I planted five rose bushes in my garden. Even though it was raining heavily, I still went out to dig them in. The soil was very heavy and wet. I had muck all over myself. It felt like I was an animal burrowing into the earth with my hands.

Colours

Argon shows an attraction to several colours, combining earthly yellows and browns with sea and sky blues to create the green of new vegetation. The orange-red of the sun is an essential contribution to plant life.

A young man in **brown** leather.

Dreamt about taking our son out as a **baby**. Put **yellow** suit on him.

Dreamt about sweets wrapped in **yellow** paper.

Dream: Wearing **yellow** gloves with 2 left hands.

Dressed baby son aged two years all **in blue** – a new outfit. I never put blue on him before now.

Attracted to a **dark blue** sweater.

Dressing up to go out, I was going to wear a **peach-coloured** blouse. But when I looked at it I decided to **wear blue**.

I feel the colour of this remedy is between **sea green** and **sky blue**, a completely **new shade of green**.

Dressed in **green** and I had a patient who was also dressed in **green**.

Dreamed of wearing **transparent green** skull caps.

Dream: woman painted with patches of **light green** paint. Colours in my life now are **yellow, brown, green, orange, blue and red**.

Can't decide on what colour paint to put on the walls of the house we are renovating. Find it hard. **Blue, yellow, orange?**

Dream: I was injecting my husband with a solution, which was **golden-orange** coloured.

Dream: **red helium** balloon rising in the distance.

Vegetation

Walking among the trees I was seeing faces, tree spirits, really friendly.

Desire for solitude to take time out to smell the flowers.

I am acutely aware of the beauty of nature. Roses blooming in November, fuchsias in full flower. Winter heather beginning to flower. A blue tit searching for berries. I can sense the energy of it all.

Dream a guest brought a flower. In it was a bug – just the legs were protruding from the bud.

Silent weeping of trees, as they are powerless to protect themselves.

There was an art exhibition on in the hotel where we went and my daughter's painting was in it. Her picture was of trees and water.

Heightened appreciation of colours and beauty. Magic swim in pool by mountain shrouded in mists, glorious with autumn colours. It is the most beautiful place in the world – but I had failed to notice the leaves had turned all last week.

Dream laying the babies on leaves.

Trees grow and fall

Trees stand at the centre of Argon, the wonderful result of nature's combined forces and the symbol of life on earth. There are several references to Christmas trees in the proving, representing the season of fun and magic for children, as well as the decorating of chopped-down trees with lights and fairies. While Argon paints the beauty of trees, it also holds the opposite, the horror of trees being felled. The vertical as opposed to horizontal aspects of this will become clear later.

I was excited at a pond surrounded by silver birches.

Felt like things were **uprighting**. I was picking up trees. The waters were fertile.

Christmas trees in red and gold!

Felt like the front of me was warm from the earth and back warm from the sun. This felt like total nourishment.

I dreamt I was in college and an old male teacher brought me back two plants. One was an evergreen Jade tree and the other one he called Gospel or Bible plant. The Gospel one had a big yellow plume like a pampas grass. I was wondering how I was going to get it to grow. It had no roots. The man laughed when I told him I had planted a lot of the green one.

Anxiety of **fallen trees**, especially when **wet**.

'Leave' – which means either to go or to produce leaves.

We had no electricity. It was Christmas Eve. We cleared the lane of fallen trees with the chainsaw we had brought with us. More and more trees blocked our way. Then the terror set in on me. I was on my own. Fear of trees coming down on top of us. Fear of not being able to get back to the children. Wondering why I had left them in the first place. It was dark and we had no lights. The roar of the wind was so bad I couldn't hear anything, not even the chain saw. All I could see in the dark were shadows. The trees were creaking and groaning and the noise was unreal. Then a tree fell on top of our car. And I wondered – what next? The fear was unreal for me, I never felt anything like this before. When we got home to the family the electricity had returned and all was normal.

Silent weeping of trees, as they are powerless to protect themselves. A quotation was sent at this time: 'Unlike white sharks, trees do not even possess the ability to defend themselves. When attacked, what arms they sometimes have – like thorns – are static, and their size and immobility mean they cannot hide. They are the most defenceless of creation in regard to man, which is why they are destroyed in such numbers'. John Fowles.

Amphibious animals

Once earth and water each occupy their own habitat, living creatures will adapt to one or the other. Argon highlights those amphibious creatures that play between both mediums, mainly the happy and playful otter, the log-like crocodile and the combination of fish and human – the magical mermaid. Boats are also a prominent feature in the proving.

Most mineral or plant remedies produce an animal analogue in their proving picture, and this animal image or behaviour may feature in cases. Helium produces eagles, Calcarea carbonica rats, Brassica platypuses, Marble cats, Belladonna dogs, Plutonium bats. It appears that the otter is one of the most prominent animals for the Argon proving.

All through the proving I have this image of being an **otter in the river**, just swimming along and enjoying myself.

Otters are semi-aquatic mammals that feed on fish and shellfish, invertebrates, amphibians, birds and small mammals. Otters are playful animals and appear to engage in behaviours, such as sliding and non-aggressive wrestling bouts, for sheer enjoyment. Otter play is pleasurable but useful, helping them to develop skills to survive in their varied environments.

The beautiful, free-flowing, swirling movement of the otter is what I am aware of. It is a scene along a riverbank with the mist of the surrounding bog and woodland all about me. There is a sense of freedom; of being allowed to do what I wish, with a clear straight river ahead, an unobstructed passage.

Went to the library to get three books about Gavin Maxwell and the otters. I have to know more about this particular life. The irreconcilableness of civilisation and culture with wildness.

Otters continue to be my strongest image representing this proving. Another prover has brought this out independently of me. I feel delighted by this. She's a perfect picture of an otter.

Other animals appear in Argon as well, mostly amphibious that bridge earth and water.

The **crocodiles'** habitat is threatened by the **destruction of trees**. They look like **floating logs**.

Anxiety for self and daughter that I wouldn't be there on her birthday – like **crocodiles** need to be present at birth.

Dream walking inside a **crocodile**.

Waking dream: I was told it was an honour for Man to fall into the Nile and be eaten by a **crocodile**. I was told crocodiles are good because they eat rough (both not smooth and not good quality) **fish**.

The 'A' horizontally felt like the open mouth of a **crocodile**.

Delusion that I was a **mermaid**.

Desire to be communicating under water.

Ears feel as if deeply **submerged**.

ALLINEATE – regulate by a line. **Amphibious craft**. Alliterate.

Dream of my husband **sailing** our family around the house at high speeds. Even though it was a **speed boat**, I didn't disapprove and I thought I might take it myself down to the water. It seemed normal the **house was full of water**.

Dream of a **Belgian** being driven out to sea in a **fast boat**. During the proving I met many Belgians.

Dream I'm on Sealink boat.

Dream I'm going in a **boat to Holland**.

Both Holland and Belgium have significant land areas that lie below sea level.

Sperm and tail

A common characteristic of amphibians is the importance of the tail. The mermaid, the crocodile and the otter all have prominent tails. While most animals possess a tail, the emphasis in amphibians is its function for maneuverability and propulsion under water and for balance on land.

There is one particular organism whose tail helps drive it over long distances – human sperm, our seed, swimming upstream in search of its Neon ovum. Seed is mentioned four times in the biblical account of the third day.

And God said: 'Let the earth put forth grass, herb yielding **seed**, and fruit-tree bearing fruit after its kind, wherein is the **seed** thereof, upon the earth.' And it was so. And the earth brought forth grass, herb yielding **seed** after its kind, and tree bearing fruit, wherein is the **seed** thereof, after its kind; . . .[4]

We have lost the **power of a tail**, it is only our human **sperm that have tails now**. A tail gives extra balance, propulsion and protection.
The letter 'a' is just an 'o' with a tail, which felt wonderful.
Is it a **fairy tale** or a **fairy tail** which is being told?
Delusion – I've got as much below my coccyx as above.
Dream collecting hen boxes, there were huge amounts of eggs.

And from Neon, waiting patiently,

Felt like one of thousands of ova sitting there waiting, with the thought that they were all female. Felt like they were there, complete and un-fertilised.

Plant evolution

Plant reproduction, namely fruits and seeds, are a major aspect of the biblical account of the third day. The vegetative life that developed on the third day used primitive forms of reproduction, asexual cell division, mitosis, and the spread of seed cells (pollen) by wind and water. Single cell organisms, such as bacteria and early algae, relied on mitosis, making identical copies, to procreate. The first organisms used the earth's heat and sulphur springs as energy sources to evolve into plants, only later learning to use solar energy through photosynthesis.

Algae evolved further by means of sexual reproduction based on haploid cells, sperm and egg cells. As life evolved within water, sperm were able to swim to the egg. Initial plants, such as bryophytes (i.e. moss, also known as pioneer plants), used water and rain in their environment as a medium and conduct for sexual reproduction. The diversity that resulted from sexual reproduction enabled plants to invade land. In order to accomplish this feat many adaptation strategies to prevent plants from drying out were required, such as the development of roots and cuticle protective coverings for the plants and "ovaries" to protect the fertilization process. Ovaries will be the base for the later development of "fruits".

More developed plants such as ferns and conifers (though primitive from a land perspective) learned to use wind as a carrier for the sperm cells (now called pollen). So, with their quantity and proximity to each other, the grasses that developed on the third day did not need to be cross-fertilized by insects. Even though fruits are mentioned in the biblical passage, they were not the result of insect fertilization but are merely a method of preserving seeds during periods of dryness.

Only at much later stages of evolution did plants begin to use insects and animals as agents for spreading their pollen and seeds. This advanced group, which we name flowering plants evolved slowly and appear in fossils from 130 million years ago. Flowers developed as an advertisement, or invitation, for insects to have sex.

The primitive flowers of Day Three, however, did not require pollination by insects or animals. Much like the naïve adolescent love displayed in Argon, early plant sexual reproduction occurred through simplistic means. It is only much later, on the fifth day, that insects and animals were created and long-distance propagation evolved through them. Perhaps the adult, loveless and advertised world of **sex** will only develop in the **Xenon** era, together with long-distance communication and city life, which evolve in the fifth period.

Dream that everything was alright because there **would be enough insects**.

During meditation feeling as if I'm **inside a chrysalis** and about to burst forth. A beautiful feeling.

Weird dream of **finding insects** which looked like the outline of a monkey. They were connected to each other by a web and the web was round a **lamp shade**.

Dream a guest brought a flower. In it was a bug – just the legs were protruding from the bud.

Buried in earth – Preservation

I was grateful that I did not rust.

The words 'preservation' and 'protection' seemed to be significant.

Feels like a warm moist void, yet no corrosion.

I was galvanizing, so that I wouldn't rust. Our thoughts untarnished. Galvanized is protective, like the difference between straight and crooked. Any action that comes from there is true, because there is no rusting.

Dream of women who were seemingly too old giving birth.

Argon is the ultimate preservative (see Chapter 2 Argon the element). Throughout the proving the theme of preservation comes up repeatedly. Before the third day there was only water; nothing could be preserved. Oxygen, the mother of life and decay, had access to all things. Once earth appears, things can be preserved, protected from the corrosive oxygen.

Earth, like Argon and salt, is a preservative. Likewise, a seed must bide its time under the earth for months and years before liberation by water. The theme of burial under the earth is prominent in the Argon proving.

An image of a corpse in a bog, being preserved for thousands of years. I was coughing up dirt from being **buried alive**.

Salt is the great preserver, which is also apparent in the picture of Natrum muriaticum. Yet Natrum muriaticum is only an imitation of its role model Argon. Natrum muriaticum preserves the negative memories of life, the disappointments, while Argon clings to the moment of perfection, the preservation of teenage love and heroism in all its glory, protected from any long-term consequence or decay. Here is the Argon thought:

Anxiety that things would rust. It stops you shining if you rust. If I do not corrode I am not responsible.

Another take on the theme of preservation is that time is only born in the fourth period; hence decay, which depends on time, is not yet possible.

Lights off

The following proving experiences all show a curious association between several elements of Argon and Day Three: earth, water, vegetation, trees, teenagers and light bulbs. Perhaps the flow of electricity through a light bulb is symbolic of the flow of life, when all these elements combine to produce the electric current of life. Contrary to this, lights go out as trees fall. No light, no shadow. Key words are in bold.

Electricity went out due to storm damage, very high winds. There were a lot of **uprooted trees**, they had come down within the past 24 hours, we had to climb over large **mature trees** to reach a clearing, when we got there we just stood still. I felt as if I was in the middle of the storm, it was **exhilarating**, didn't feel afraid even though there were **trees falling around us.**

I heard noisy **teenagers** outside and became frightened. Got out of bed and tried to turn on the **lights, they didn't work,** went into my mother's, **her lights didn't work** either. Looked out a window, it was like dawn, saw a female neighbour shoving **earth** from a truck into another garden and thought that was the reason the **lights wouldn't come on.**

Dream an old friend from childhood was there and kept **turning out the lights,** which annoyed me. We moved outside to the **sea front** and were walking and dancing along. I went out in front, a young man in a

brown leather jacket started to follow, got scared as I knew he wasn't part of the group.

Summary

Day Three of creation in the Bible tells two stories, first of the separation of water from earth and then of their interplay resulting in first life. The proving of Neon relates to the first half, where earth is concealed within water, and hence there is water everywhere. The proving of Argon tells the story of the second half, of earth and water flirting, playing and frolicking and finally producing seed and flower.

Argon is element 18. According to Jewish numerology (*Gimatria*) 18 signifies the word 'Chai', which means life. Day Three of creation depicts evolution from the inanimate into life. While Neon prepares the waters, the ground is not yet ready for growth. After the waters pull back to expose the earth and land and sea separate, the relationship between the two can begin; blue seas evaporate and condense to green rivers, which irrigate the yellow earth. Seeds are sown, grasses grow, trees seek sun, otters and mermaids play on the shore. New life dances, sings and laughs in the magical garden of creation; the world is in bloom.

And it was good.

Postscript: The Sabbath

As with the other nobles, Argon also represents the noble seventh day, the Sabbath, a day when all is peaceful and perfect, without interaction with the external world of toil and work.

Everything seems amazingly easy, so smooth, like I rested on the 7th day. It is the seven days repeated seven times, a bigger cycle.

From this we learn that every noble is a Sabbath, the day of rest. Seven times seven, is the cycle of 7 nobles or Sabbaths, each with its individual flavor.[i]

---

[i] In Judaism the cycle of Seven Sabbaths occurs between Passover and the festival of Shavuot.

Except from *Song of the Broad-Axe* (1900) by American poet and journalist Walter (Walt) Whitman (1819–1882):

Welcome are all earth's lands, each for its kind,
Welcome are lands of pine and oak,
Welcome are lands of the lemon and fig,
Welcome are lands of gold,
Welcome are lands of wheat and maize – welcome those of the grape,
Welcome are lands of sugar and rice,

Welcome the cotton-lands – welcome those of the white potato and sweet
  potato,
Welcome are mountains, flats, sands, forests, prairies,
Welcome the rich borders of rivers, table-lands, openings,
Welcome the measureless grazing lands – welcome the teeming soil of orchards,
  flax, honey, hemp,
Welcome just as much the other more hard-faced lands,
Lands rich as lands of gold, or wheat and fruit lands,
Lands of mines, lands of the manly and rugged ores,
Lands of coal, copper, lead, tin, zinc,
Lands of iron! lands of the make of the axe![5]

References

1   Genesis 1:9–13. Available online at: https://biblia.com/bible/esv/Ge1.9–13
2   Who was Korach? Available online at: http://www.chabad.org/parshah/article_cdo/aid/45961/jewish/Who-Was-Korach.htm
3   Genesis 8:5–7 Available online at: https://biblia.com/bible/Genesis8
4   Genesis 1:11–12 Available online at: https://biblia.com/books/esv/Ge1.11
5   Whitman W. Song of the Broad-Axe. In: *Leaves of Grass*. New York: Signet Classics/Penguin Group USA (Special edn), 2005. Available online at: https://tinyurl.com/y7do3by8

9

ARGON MEDITATION PROVING

The following is a meditation proving done by my wife Camilla, by holding the remedy. *Camilla had no idea what the remedy was.* She is, however, very talented at producing quick, accurate and useful remedy pictures.

You may be of the 'science excludes all' branch of homoeopathy, and consider meditation provings an abomination. Take it or leave it, what you don't know won't hurt you (usually). The important thing is that this proving stands alongside a full, comprehensive Hahnemannian proving and not as a stand-alone. (See Chapter 14, *Meditation provings* for fuller explanation.)

The proving was recorded verbatim from the moment it began.

(Observation) Immediately smiling and laughing.

I'm possessed.

Hey – we are allowed to drink! We are adults! We can drink and smoke and stay up all night and no one will tell us to stop! Ha-ha! Like we don't need permission from mummy any more. Ha!

Carefree, happy and drink? No one can tell us what to do. There are no adults. We are the adults but not really, ha-ha!

This feels like America – first year university – drink and smoke and bonk (have sex) in my room. I'm in America; I can feel my accent changing. I feel like the young girl in the movie *The Graduate*.[i] A first taste of freedom – fresh freedom. No one will tell us it is bedtime or that we have to get up. You are your own boss and you can do what and whatever you want. It is accepted and expected.

I can do anything I want, the world is my apple! I rule with my youth ... I'm 21, no, I'm 19, 18 even. You do because you can! It is your birth right and no one can stop you. It's not even a rebellion; it is what comes naturally at that age. Like going overseas when you finish high school. Young and free, it's expected and you can, and oh my God it's so good! No care in the world, fees paid. Comfort and luxury, future secured. You know you will marry someone rich just like you. You are from the privileged line

---
[i] 1967 film *The Graduate* (United Artists).

– like the Kennedys. Inherited money, the people that rule, tradition. All fun and easy, a thin veneer, no real issues, like not being told to go to bed. But good fun. On the holidays you go home to your rich family's house, Thanksgiving and eggnog, little issues – ha-ha-ha, who cares! Storms in a teacup.

(Observation) She begins cheerfully singing the song *Mrs. Robinson*[i] from the movie *The Graduate*.

God doesn't come into this, not God's grace or anything. God does not feature in the credits of this movie – 'Busy elsewhere'. Ha-ha.

You marry someone that fits the part, a pre-set husband, pre-set life and kids, and they do the same. Big Christmas trees, pudding, your birth-right. Now you are free. Mummy won't tell you to go to bed or get up, you are 18.

First time out, first taste of freedom. This is naive and innocent, not hard core. You are still expected to be in the framework though. Like Mrs. Robinson. She wants to be like her daughter. Feels like Berkeley, California, undergraduate, young person in first year in university, carefree, sunshine. This is so shallow and unreal, skin-deep but with tradition. Like old money and telling stories of how it was when you were a kid in a rich home; Christmas trees in red and gold!

Innocent remedy, you are still a kid but you grew up.

18 years old, just out of home, not even a graduate. But the problem is you never really grow up, you are stuck in the pattern. It becomes a tradition. Never change, just more, more, more of the same. Like the Kennedys. The only way out is to be killed young. This remedy cannot mature – it can only repeat itself, hence the tradition.

Nowhere to go from here. How much can you get out of it . . . cool at 18, but at 63. . . . This is boring. It was fun at the beginning, but after a while. . . . It's fun to look like a baby doll at 18, but at 54? Having a face lift. Looking like 54 on outside but inside 18. Pathetic.

There is a time and a place for everything. In this remedy time and space have stopped, this remedy is stuck like a broken record. (Singing: *'Doo doo doo doo, Mrs. Robinson, every way you look you look at it you lose')*.[i] Like someone who never realised that time moved on. Like Mrs. Robinson – The boredom of it.

This remedy feels like Krypton (She was one of the Krypton provers – JS) – repetition of time. But Krypton was much more difficult, everything stuck and a nightmare, here everything is so shallow.

---

[i] From the song *Mrs Robinson* (Columbia) recorded by Simon and Garfunkel in 1968

To get yourself out of this repetition you would have to shake yourself like a wet dog. Do a lot of yoga and drink health juice and all that new age bullshit. Ha-ha. The only way out is self-realisation, need to wake up and realise yourself. You got to choose. (Singing *'Every way you look at it you choose'* from the song *Mrs. Robinson.*)

This remedy is like the 60's. You could do anything – you could fuck without getting pregnant – the ultimate freedom! Frivolous. Old money with tradition. Seems like West coast more than East coast. They don't want change, want to be mummy and daddy's girl forever, only with a bit of freedom. Repeat the cycle. This remedy can lead to addiction and alcoholism, depression. Resisting change. I feel this remedy is before Scandium (She was a prover of Scandium – JS). They can't even try to make a choice.

(Still singing *Mrs Robinson* 'Where *have you* gone Joe DiMaggio'.) Like an old baseball player – you want to keep the same but the magic has gone. Nothing lives up to the way it was. Hey, Paul Simon is a genius. The song that came up for the Krypton proving was *Slip Sliding Away* and now this song. How did he move from one to the other? (She still does not know what the remedy is – JS). There is blindness in this remedy, a tunnel vision.

Comment

I regard this as a remarkable and clinically useful proving. The connection between Argon, element 18, and the coming of age at eighteen years tells us much about the nature of this remedy. While there is initial joy at the freedom, competence and privilege of mature youth, it is the attempt to hold on to this peak moment of existence that causes the pathology to manifest. Argon is a preservative, but preserving our youth cannot revive its charm. Fun turns to boredom, play into chore, joy into an addiction to cheap thrills. Argon attempts to preserve to the last remnants of a magical childhood; perhaps the best of it – youth – the playfulness of childhood mixed with the freedom and capability of an 18-year-old. But even Peter Pan must eventually grow up and become a productive adult. There is a shadow side waiting to emerge, and we cannot lose it forever.

The image of privileged and rich tradition that arises in this proving serves to enhance the golden moment of youth. Not only are we in the prime of life, but there is no need to work or take early responsibility. Dustin Hoffman in *The Graduate* returns from college to an empty life, with no responsibilities and no joy; an inert limbo between childhood and adulthood.

Are we responsible for another when we are 18, are we responsible at 18?

The ageing Mrs. Robinson seeks to regain some of her lost youth through him, but this tastes empty. His only solution is to seek perfect love with her daughter Elaine, and the movie ends in the golden moment of their elopement. But what happens next? Where will they live, what will they do, will they have kids, a mortgage, responsibilities and problems? Who cares! We are left with the image of the glowing young couple at the back of the bus.

It is interesting to note the connection to the other nobles in this meditation proving – Krypton and Xenon (element 54). For some reason Paul Simon songs feature in the other nobles; Neon (*Sound of Silence*), Argon (*Mrs. Robinson*) and Krypton (*Slip Sliding Away*).

Notice the reference to Christmas trees. The theme of trees is a major aspect of Argon, and the Christmas tree symbolises a tree at its most glorious moment. This appearance is deceptive. Like a middle-aged person trying to cling to youth, the tree is cut from its roots. The joy is artificial.

10

ARGON 50M SENSATION, FUNCTION, STRUCTURE

We now leave the realm of affinities and emotions, nouns and adjectives, and move to the realm of sensation and function, which deal with the position and movement of bodies in time and space. Functions, or verbs, represent the motion of the vital force as mediated by the nervous system. We sense the environment and respond with a function.

The following symptoms are accounts from different provers that show a remarkable consistency in regards to motion in space. The themes are simple and need no explanation, though later we will learn how the totality of these concepts weave into one idea consistent with the inner nature of Argon.

We begin with the vertical alignment of Argon. In the previous books of this series we perceived a recurring theme running through the noble gases. The central axis of life is a vertical line extending from centre heaven to mid-earth, with which the noble gases align in a state of health or misalign in disease.[i] When in line with this axis, energy can flow and the vital force is galvanised with universal current.

As in the preceding nobles, Helium and Neon, Argon is aligned with this upright axis of life and truth, here and now.

Aligned

Feeling in **complete alignment**, settled in the middle of my soul, body and emotions. I feel **taller**.

I feel **above it all**, looking down on the wonderful world. Feel as if I could fly.

---

[i] See Angles of the Periodic Table in Sherr, J. *A Dynamic Materia Medica of The Noble Gases: Neon*. Glasgow: Saltire Books, 2016, pp55–8.

Felt like things were **uprighting**. I was **picking up** trees.

Felt like the sun was always shining, granting power to be and to act. Also about **angles and the shadow warps us**, and the size of the shadow is in direct relation to **our angle**, our relationship to the sun. If the sun is **directly above**, there's no shadow.

Understanding – two pillars are mutually supportive and when they're **vertical**.

ALLINEATE – **regulate by a line**. Amphibious craft. Alliterate.

Aware that the truth is **straight**, deceit is **crooked**.

Sensation that I was **lying** waiting, like I was **horizontal** lying but not telling lies lying.

Whatever you are is right for you. It's all a bit **convoluted**. This feeling of things being in the **right order** fit me **back into place**. I had been jolted **out of place**.

Obstruction

Dream, driving down the motorway, saw an articulated lorry across both lanes.

Things keep happening. Driving cars seemed to come at us from every corner. Sometimes it seemed absurdly tricky, other times unremarkable and I didn't even slow down.

Thought we were closer to side of road, like the road was narrower and closing in.

Backed out of the parking lot into another car. I didn't even see the other car.

Desire to drive faster, more careless driving, braking too fast, skidding, near-misses.

Felt frustrated, communication seems to be delayed, cheques, post, etc. Felt I wasted time. Lots of delays in different situations.

Dream of a woman in a red mini crashing into things, and a woman in a white mini who was very angry about it. I asked her why she did not reverse and she said, "There is no true reverse."

Missed a flight today because I didn't give myself enough time. Normally I would always find a way. The girl at the desk would not let me through. I was soon angry and fighting with everyone. No one wanted to help. The girl was completely unmoved, as if she felt I had done it on purpose. People were completely unbudgeable. I couldn't change things. When I was looking to people for help I was coming up against brick walls.

Feels like I shouldn't be restricted in any way – like in society. Insisting I was right in a situation where I wasn't. Wanting to get my own way.

Left home with Andy to get gas as the power was gone due to the storm and we had no electricity. It was Christmas Eve. We cleared the lane (driveway to our house) of fallen trees with the chainsaw we had brought with us. The first thing we meet on the road was a galvanised roof, which had blown off one of our sheds. Then more and more trees blocked our way. I was on my own – separated from Andy and the children who were at home alone. Fear of trees coming down on top of us. Fear of Andy not being able to get back. Fear of not being able to get back to the children. Wondering why I had left them in the first place. It was dark and we had no lights. I had given Andy the matches. The roar of the wind was so bad we couldn't hear anything, not even the chain saw. All I could see in the dark were shadows. The trees were creaking and groaning and the noise was unreal. Then another car came up behind me. It was a woman driving. I told her she would have to go back. She said she should have known, it was silly of her to come this way. Then a tree fell on top of our car. And I wondered – what next? The fear was unreal for me, I never felt anything like this before.

Unobstructed flow

Unbelievable **smooth easiness**.

Continuous and repeated dreams of **running**.

Dream building walls from barbed wire, enjoying it.

Totally directed in actions. A **clear path ahead; a straight line**. Unable to tolerate anyone who might stand in my way or present an obstacle to me. I feel I will beat them up or smack them out of the way. Completing one goal and then **moving on** to the next one.

Dream I drove a car in a marquee and I shot through a canvas wall and then another, felt great to **drive through them** and see the shape of the car.

Better able to **get through** jobs hanging over me. Cleared things that had been overwhelming and were tormenting me. Very focused and methodical, achieving things that didn't seem achievable.

Completing tasks quickly and finally getting things done. Feel I am catching up on lost time and **moving on**.

Feeling of clarity of thought and of deep connection. Energy very high and focused. **Feeling of flowing**.

I felt like going with the flow. Adapting to everything much more softly. **I do not feel the sharp and stinging resistance**, the disruptive edges anymore.

Leave hospital very late – extremely satisfied with my work. I had felt all day **'like being carried by wings'** – floating through hospital corridors, felt high and alert.

There was a great sense of energy, a surge of energy to complete tasks and objectives. There was a sense of having a great deal of power behind me, a huge support. Something was **pushing me forward and there was no going back**.

All through the proving I have this image of being an otter in the river, just swimming along and enjoying myself. The beautiful, free-flowing, swirling movement of the otter is what I am aware of. It is a scene along a river bank with the mist of the surrounding bog and woodland all about me. There is a sense of freedom; of being allowed to do what I wish, with a clear straight river ahead: **an unobstructed passage**.

The driving experience is quite pleasurable with **freedom of movement on the road**.

This is my life's pattern – **the harder I run, the further I get behind**. I know what to do and not to do but it doesn't help – I can't work like other people. Very slowly the right course is coming to light.

Instead of feeling in a fog of tiredness, I have an urge to **get up and go** to the pool to swim before everyone else surfaces.

Extremely productive day – backlog of organising various things finished – more than I would often get done.

Very focused and methodical in what I'm doing, get **more done** in one hour than I would normally get done in a half day.

Very organised today compared to how cloudy I was feeling yesterday. Getting things done quickly. Doing what needs to be done. Move the house around. **Moving the furniture to open the space up**.

Easy travel

Travel seems very easy.

Travel again easy today and what could have turned out to be very difficult crossing was in fact **plain sailing**.

Speed

I was a passenger in a friend's car and even though we were doing 50–60mph I felt it was only about 30mph and wanted him to go faster.

Sensation that we were **travelling faster** than we were, checked speedometer, 40mph.

Connection

Husband phoned me – was very surprised, really thrilled, couldn't believe it, felt **connected again**.

Very happy when supervisor rang – felt **connected again**.

Extraordinary sense of connection growing within the group all through college weekend.

Feeling of ease and contentment – **connected** to the Universe, the Earth, the Sea.

Feeling of clarity of thought and of **deep connection**.

Thoughts of connection/connectedness.

Felt **connected** to earth and spirit. Sense of oneness, as if I would dissolve into energy of waves, sea, sand, sky.

Felt **completely connected** to my husband when he held me. Wanted to make love with him.

Great **love and connectedness** with grandparents. Felt like crying with happiness.

Started dancing to radio music. Feel **very connected** – and light hearted.

Desire for connection. I had a strong desire to phone friends. I rang four friends . . . they usually phone me so it was strange for me to have this **desire to make contact**.

Misconnection

Dropped phone into mug of tea prior to leaving the country for a week, thus making communication difficult.

Communication difficult today because phone messages are misunderstood.

I have managed to leave my phone behind when I travelled yesterday.

Disconnected feeling, not quite here.

I had lost the feeling of completeness and connectedness. There is a big empty void inside me. I am a walking corpse.

Assertive

I normally get my **own way** more subtly, now I am more **assertive**.

Desire to go out. **I insisted on going out**. I was a right bitch, wanted my **own way**. Normally, I wouldn't bother. I wanted to dress up and **get out there**.

Feel decisive – a new determination has now crystallised or more like cemented. In fact, I think I am hardening up. I can see that **struggling is always futile**.

Felt more assertive at work, didn't feel I had to get angry to **make my point**.

Assertive with people, letting them know exactly what is required. Completing tasks quickly and finally getting things done. Feel I am **catching up** on lost time and **moving on**.

Sharper with people, blunt and **direct**, confronting people.

Summary

We have learnt that Argon is capable of two extremes. On one hand there is an obstructed and difficult passage through life, where every road and avenue seems blocked. This was very much my experience during the proving, when a pleasant 'should be two-hours' journey though Ireland turned into an eight-hour, obstructed nightmare. This sense of frustrated effort is associated with a feeling of disconnection. Conversely, there is a sense of unobstructed free flow, ease of travel, effortless achievement and assertive forward movement. These are associated with a sense of connection. The sense of connection or lack of connection reminds us that Argon is associated with the third chakra (or fifth chakra if counting from the bottom up) that represents the throat and communication. Argon also relates to sperm, so we might speculate that it could be a good remedy in infertility, especially from obstructed passageways.

The factor that decides which of these two paths we will travel is our alignment with the source of life, much as we saw in Neon and Helium. Either we are aligned and flowing or we are misaligned and impeded. When the sun is directly above there is no shadow to obscure and obstruct our journey through life. The current of noble universal energy flows through us and turns on our light.

Feeling in **complete alignment**, settled in the **middle of** my soul, body and emotions. I feel taller.

Felt like the sun was always shining, granting power to **be and to act**. Also about **angles and the shadow warps us**, and the size of the shadow is in direct relation to **our angle**, our relationship to the sun. If the sun is **directly above, there's no shadow**.

Woke with a feeling of bleakness, a sense of hopelessness and **lack of direction** in my life. A feeling I don't know where **my place is in life**. Felt **better when I got up**. More into accepting whatever is right for now. **Whatever you are is right for you**. It's all a bit convoluted. This feeling of things being in the right order fit me back into place. I had been **jolted out of place**.

Even when I was disorientated, I was slipping but correcting – as though I had an amazing self-correcting mechanism.

Day Three Argon

Our lights were on
Now they are-gone,
We're out of line
The sun don't shine.

Our angle bent
Shade descent,
Obscuring joy
With discontent.

The sea will not
Convert to cloud,
Rain won't fall
Plants won't thrive.

Rivers will not
Flow to sea,
Trees fall down
T'ween you and me.

Our path is blocked
Get nothing done,
Our youth is lost
No childhood fun.

If only we
Could stand upright,
Open throat
Reclaim birthright.

Our light to shine
Our love to flow,
Youth to blossom
Tree to grow.

11

ARGON CM NEW DIMENSIONS

Two to three

On our journey down the periodic table we have moved from the second to the third noble gas. Below are some of the symptoms that illustrate the transition from two to three. Note the references to flat water before it retracts from land.

Bought three fish but only two people. Felt there should be a third.

Dream I am in bed, near my feet is a glass bottle of mineral water. I push it with my feet, it fell on the carpet. There was **water all over the carpet**. There were **three** nice glasses and the bottle fell on them, the glasses broke. I went downstairs and saw **two** dead pigs on the table.

I dreamt I was swimming in the **ocean** with **two men**. There were **large waves** and a **strong tide** – it was thrilling. I then ran **along the road beside the sea** in my blue swimsuit.

Dream of pushing **two beds** together, bottom to head, not side by side, a **man and a woman** got into one and **myself** into the other.

Dream of **two people** coughing up blood and appear to be wounded. They are both on their knees and are dying. **Another person** runs to get help.

Dream **two men** on bicycles, dressed in black, were going to be knocked down by a big red bus.

Dream of expecting an inspection by **two** women. My **three** sisters-in-law were there and being lazy.

Felt very good, the **three of us** together (self and two daughters).

Dimensions

In the previous books of this series we discovered that the physical dimensions unfold in parallel to the periodic table, reaching the peak of each dimension at the noble gas. This understanding is extremely important as well as clinically useful.

We may say that pre-Hydrogen is a non-dimensional state (or perhaps a tenth or eleventh dimensional state[i]), a non-element, which playfully can be called Nononium. This no-thing concentrates into a pre-dimension, a dot or singularity. The dot explodes in all directions, which results in a state of no boundaries – Hydrogen. Helium's reaction is to concentrate this amorphous cosmic soup into the first dimension, a line (as in light's linear state[ii]). The second period and Neon spread this line into the second dimension of surface. We have learnt that Neon is analogous to 'super-water', having the same number of electrons as H_2O. Water always finds its own level and is therefore flat; hence Neon exists in a superficial flatland. Argon unfolds the third dimension, space, which can be measured by volume. In the next book of this series we will observe Krypton concentrating time into a line.

With each extra dimension, we evolve, we get more room to maneuver, yet we are restricted by the new dimension's characteristics. Helium enjoys the freedom of a soul without a body, but is confined to a one-dimensional line: To be or not to be, to remain body-less or to descend to earth. In the Helium patient this linear tendency may manifest as repetitive thoughts or OCD. Neon is confined to a two-dimensional surface, occupied with infantile superficial desires, which may develop into addictions. The third dimension of volume or space evolves in Argon. Before this dimension is fully unfolded, motion is restricted and a sense of obstruction is apparent. As the third dimension fully opens, Argon can flow freely. The proving clearly exhibits these extremes: obstruction versus free flow on the physical, mental and emotional planes.

One should be clear about the difference between dimension and direction (Figure 11.1). Direction is the attitude of a line: north-south, east-west or up-down. It makes no difference to the dimensions what axis each of the three lines lies on. It is the combination of one, two or three lines placed at 90^0 to each other that forms the first three dimensions. When a length develops a perpendicular width, it becomes surface. When a surface develops a perpendicular height/depth it becomes volume.

---

[i] To better understand the Tenth Dimension, see the video, *Imagining the Tenth Dimension* R. Bryanton. Available online at https://www.youtube.com/watch?v=8Q_GQqUg6Ts

[ii] See Alternative Dimensions. In: Sherr J. *A Dynamic Materia Medica of the Noble Gases: Neon.* Glasgow: Saltire Books, 2016. pp208–12.

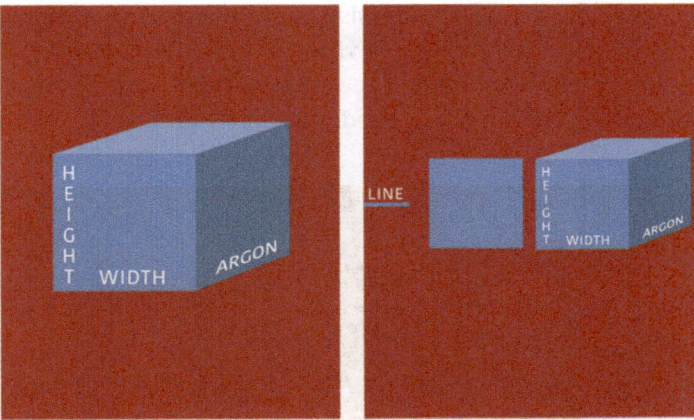

Figure 11.1 *Directions and dimensions*

A line placed in any direction is one-dimensional, a surface in any direction is still two-dimensional, and a cube in any direction is three dimensional.

The development of the third dimension in Argon may be seen either as gaining height or breadth, depending on one's orientation in space. The proving depicts both aspects, with some symptoms showing Argon as developing breadth (Figure 11.2 left side), while other symptoms show Argon developing height (Figure 11.2 right side).

Which one should we chose? The answer is both. Argon extends into breadth to make wider corridors with easier passage (Figure 11.2 left side).

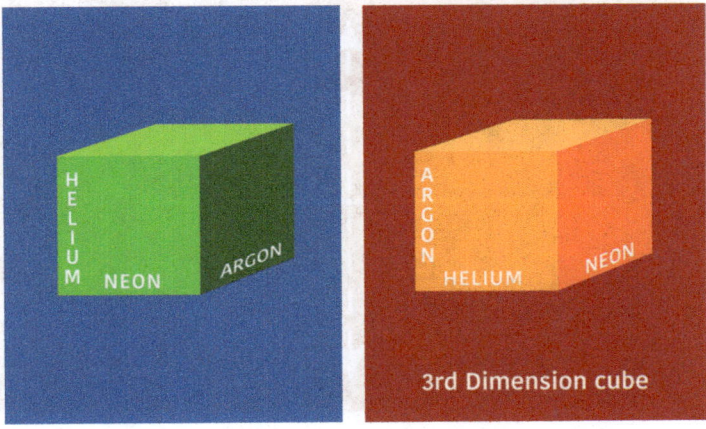

Figure 11.2 *Two different views of the direction of the three dimensions and the related noble gases. Argon may be viewed as representing height or breadth*

However, since the proving emphasises more symptoms of Argon lending height, we will concentrate on this viewpoint (Figure 11.2 right side).

We begin in the beginning: The universe starts with a singularity in which all dimensions are compressed into one (Figure 11.3).

Figure 11.3 All dimensions in one, singularity

Helium develops the first dimension of line. We may view this line as either vertical or horizontal (Figure 11.4). When laid horizontally Helium represents the separation of the higher spiritual world from the lower world of physical manifestation. The Helium patient is often stuck between these two states.

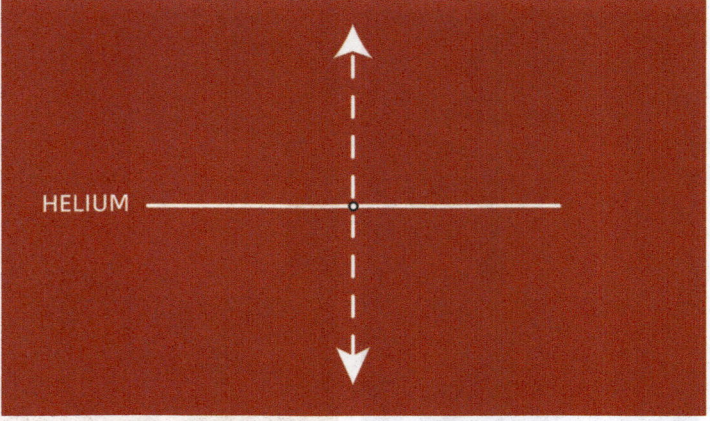

Figure 11.4 Helium extends the dot into a line that separates the world into above and below

Helium is trapped in its line. To free itself, it must stretch into a new dimension – surface. Helium splits horizontally into two as it progresses through the second period and the second day of creation (Figure 11.5).

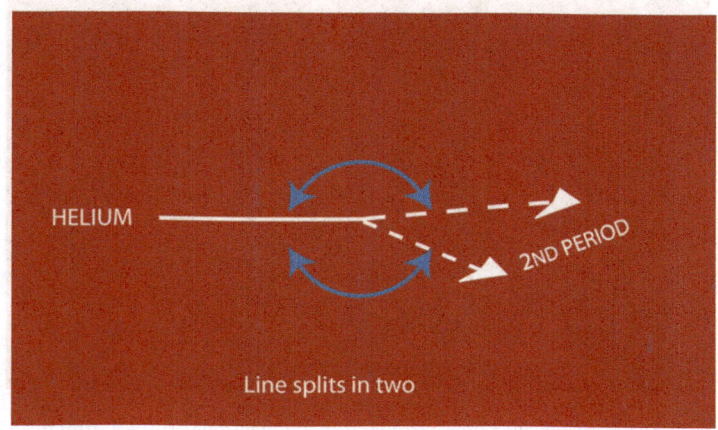

Figure 11.5 *Helium's line splitting horizontally*

Once the split has fully manifested, a new direction is created – width (Figure 11.6).

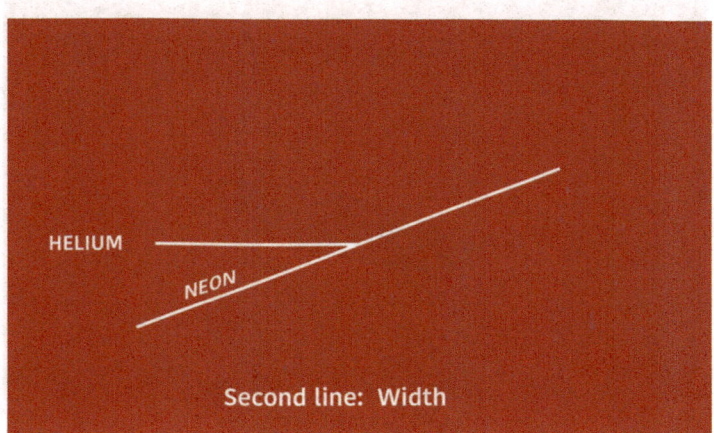

Figure 11.6 *Line has split and created a new perpendicular line within a plane*

The combination of both of these lines, length and width, creates a two-dimensional surface, a firmament (Figure 11.7).

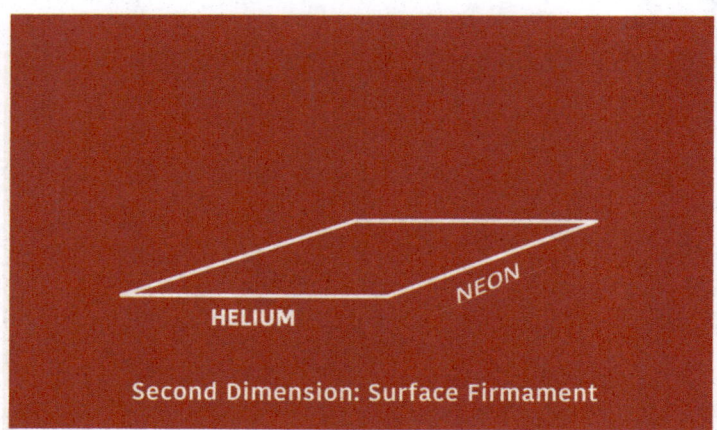

Second Dimension: Surface Firmament

Figure 11.7 Two perpendicular lines creating a two-dimensional surface; firmament

At this stage of creation water is spread over the surface of the earth – as in Day Two of creation (Figure 11.8).

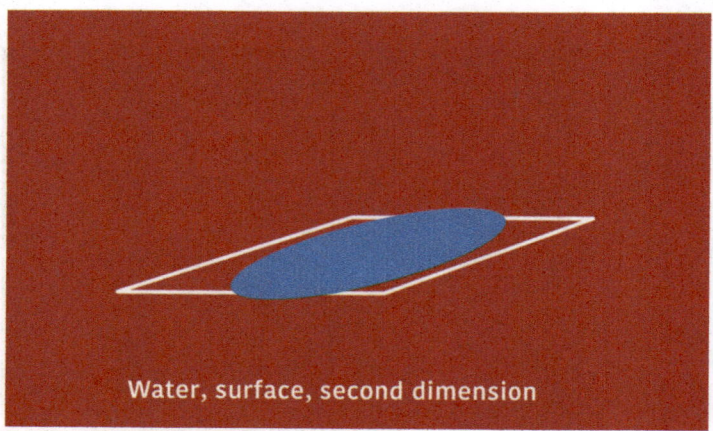

Water, surface, second dimension

Figure 11.8 Water as earth's surface

In the beginning of Day Three, water collects to one spot (Figure 11.9). It does this by spinning inwards as a helix or whirlpool. Land is uncovered.

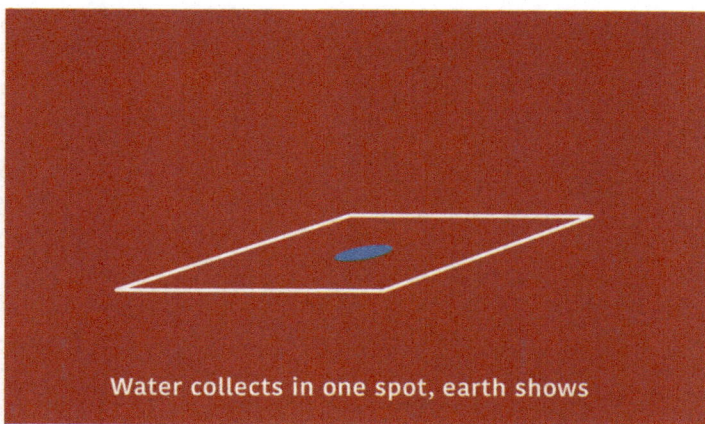

Water collects in one spot, earth shows

Figure 11.9 *Water collecting to one spot*

Because water concentrates and is no longer spread out, a third dimension begins to manifest as land rises. As water retreats, land rises (Figure 11.10).

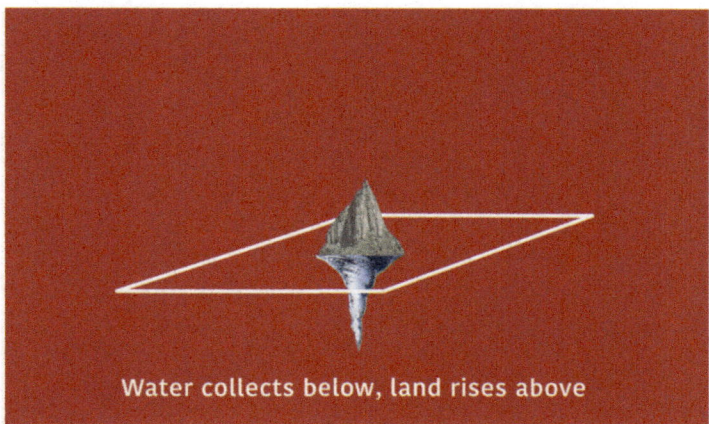

Water collects below, land rises above

Figure 11.10 *Water concentrates below as land rises*

The separation of earth and water is a first step to the third dimension, which begins to unfold as height (Figure 11.11).

I was rising up from the ocean. I could see the spray caught by the wind turning into foam. My skin was smooth and watery.

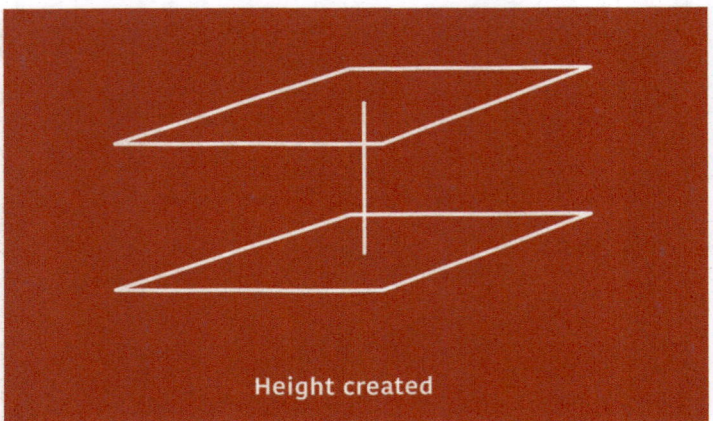

Figure 11.11 *Height creating a third dimension*

As life evolves into the third dimension and the third day of creation, water evaporates into clouds and falls as rain, roots reach downwards and trees grow skywards (Figure 11.12).

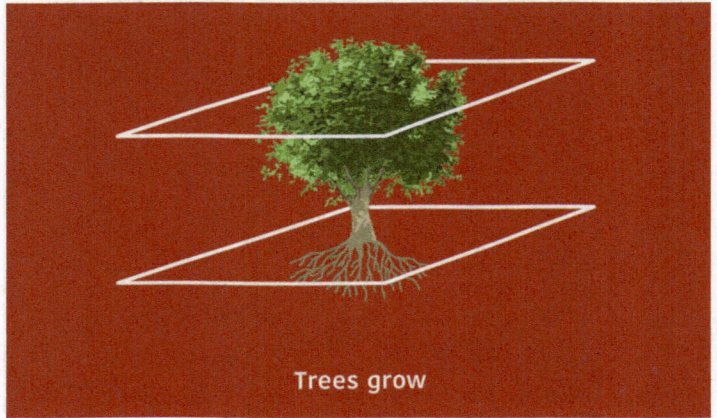

Figure 11.12 *Tree grows skywards, seeking sun and providing shade*

The following illustration (Figure 11.13) shows how each of the three axes split the world into two directions and returns us to the issue of how directions and dimensions can be viewed in multiple ways. Helium's horizontal line creates an up-down split of soul and body, Neon's width creates the forward and backwards of future and past, desire and aversion, and Argon's vertical direction creates the width of corridor or gateway for life to flow through.

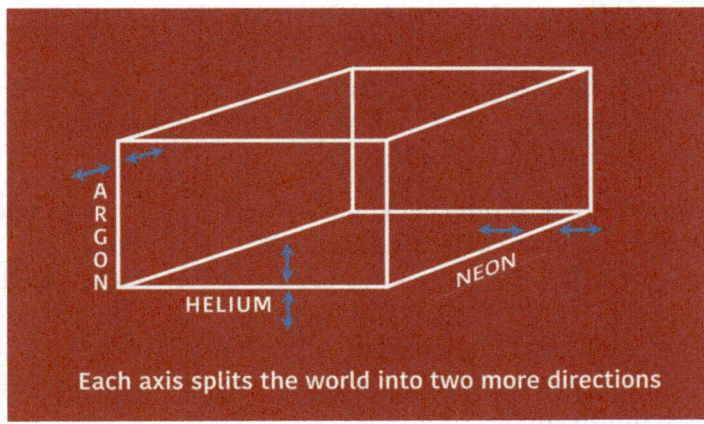

Figure 11.13 Each axis splitting the world into two more directions

Viewing the same process from another angle, we may say that the process of unfolding dimension begins from the mid-axis of our being, (Helium, first dimension, one eye), then moving forward to our two eyes (Neon, second dimension) and then to both eyes conjoined, where stereo-scopic vision forms (Argon, third dimension). In Krypton our mind will begin to circle around our frontal lobes, creating the fourth dimension of so-called 'time'.

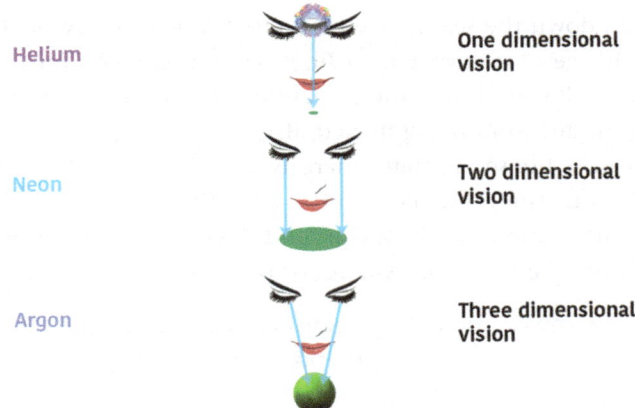

Figure 11.14 Three dimensions of vision

The third dimension unfolding in the proving

We will now compare Argon symptoms and expressions with the unfolding of the third dimension. We begin with the two-dimensional surface inherited from Neon (Figure 11.15).

Dream **two-dimensional** grey, dark, black shapes, **rectangles and triangles** in twisted wreckage like after a war.

Sensation that I was lying waiting, like I was **horizontal lying** but not telling lies lying.

People's heads appeared **flattened**.

When sitting, felt like **sitting low and slouched** in a chair and seeing in a **different direction**.

He was only seeing above the ground. He had no tail.

Maybe I am **out of my depth** here!

Cells only split when they're **horizontal**.

Thought we were closer to side of road, like the road was narrower and closing in.

Seas separate from earth, leaving a water-logged horizontal surface. Life is still buried in the earth in the form of a seed, along with the decomposing organic material needed for its growth.

Anxiety on seeing **horizontal** wet wood or **fallen trees**, especially when wet.

I pushed down the seat in the car so that it was **totally horizontal** and I had an image of a **corpse in a bog**, being **preserved** for thousands of years. The following day I was coughing and the image was that I was coughing up dirt from being **buried alive**.

Dream of a house. Upstairs there is a baby on a table. The **baby is strapped on to the table**. Behind the table there is no wall, a **big space, up to the attic**, and down to the ground floor. I was worried that the baby might **fall off the table**, but **she is strapped on**.

In the next phase the third dimension begins to unfold. The process of expanding into height involves rotation, from the horizontal to the vertical (Figure 11.15).

It feels as though my face is turning, the left side is going over to the top and the right side to the bottom, with my mouth in the centre.

Until now the lower half is hidden.

Like an iceberg, you just see the tip but there is so much more below.

I've got as much below my coccyx as above.
I kept seeing halves, half above and half below.

Now height unfurls, duplicating above what has been hidden below. This starts gradually with 9 and then 18 degrees above and below, and then unfolding to 90 degrees (Figure 11.15a). Second dimension splits and begins to unfurl the third dimension of height (compare Figure 11.5).

He said I owed him lots of money, that I could pay him just half. I said, 'No, I will double it', i.e. I would pay double what I owed.
Felt like I came out of a scallop shell. A flat egg. Half shells or whole shells. Half a shell is 9. I felt reptilian.

Note: The crocodile, which appears often in Argon, represents the flat second dimension (Figure 11.15b).

Sensation when walking that I was leaning back at an incredible angle and my feet were a long way in front of my head. I didn't know which was my back or my front, I had the delusion that my back was my front. I slipped on the mud and came back upright.
If wood is vertical and it is raining it's fine, but if horizontal it will decay.
Dreamt the cloth was removed and exposed a huge attic space, another floor.
Feels like before the serpent lost its legs.
The Milky Way is the white road, the road of awe. When the Milky Way is lying **flat, skimming the horizon**, the area overhead is completely dark. A huge door opened inwards to the left. This is the portal into which beings of **other worlds** emerge out of.
There is as much below as above. The angles need the same below and above. If it was 18 degrees below it would have to be 108. 90 + 18 = 108 (Figure 11.15c).

Now we have space to play in. If our length, width and height are fully expanded, we are provided with a wide corridor of life though which we can freely flow, achieving all that we want with ease. If, however, our dimensions are constricted we will meet with obstructions everywhere, as we collide with the edges of life's narrow passageway.

When driving I find it **hard to judge the width** of the car. As a result I drive more slowly and cautiously.
Thought we were closer to side of road, like the road was narrower.
At the airport had to run as fast as possible down **long corridor** to catch flight.
Dream of building bridges and then **crossing bridges**.

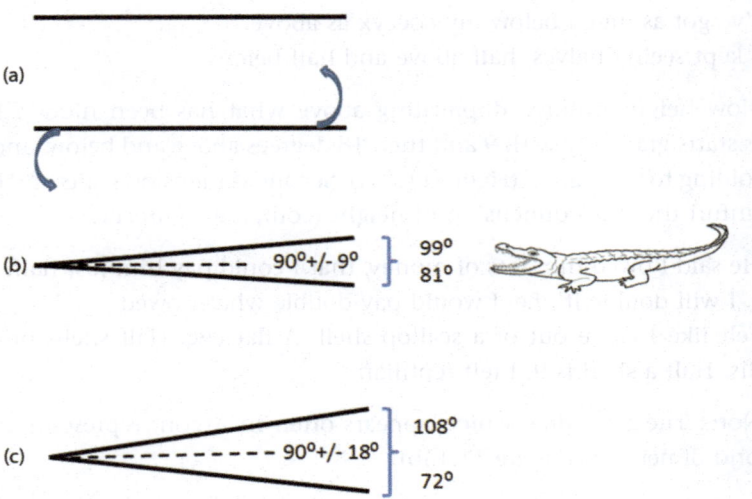

Figure 11.15a–c Unfurling of the third dimension

Dream **wedging the car into a space** in an exclusive camping place.

Driving cars seemed to come at us from every corner. Sometimes it seemed absurdly tricky, other times unremarkable and I didn't even slow down.

Desire to drive faster, more careless driving, braking too fast, skidding, near misses.

Dream I drove a car in a marquee and I shot through a canvas wall and then another, felt great to drive through them and see the shape of the car.

The following expression shows how by creating height, we also open width.

Understanding – two pillars are mutually supportive and when they're **vertical**, there's **space in between**, but when **horizontal** one has to be above the other which is a **restriction** (Figure 11.16).

When our consciousness evolves into the third dimension, so does our architecture and dreams. The world now rises into height and falls into depth.

Light bright, **height** and sight, no fight, yet I might.

Dream of a trapdoor in floor of huge room. Instead of joists there are rolled carpets the whole **length and width**.

Dream **sliding down** many huge banisters in a college library with a friend. Very fast and fun, but I went too far and ended up in the **basement**.

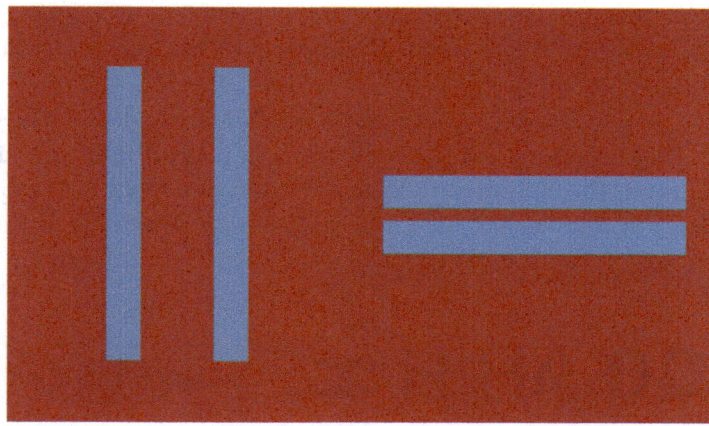

Figure 11.16 *Two vertical pillars with space between and two horizontal pillars that restrict*

Dream I was going out the **upper entrance** to avoid going through the building **downstairs**, but then I re-entered from the **ground floor**.

Dream I decided to look for my mother, saw all these older people in a file on a large **winding staircase**, my mother's friends. Felt I had to find my mother to warn her that my friends were having a party **downstairs**, went into various rooms, it was an old house and very big, I enjoyed exploring it, didn't find my mother and ended up in an orchard, where a woman was spraying the **apple trees**.

Apple trees – into this new dimension plants can grow. At this stage, we must ask ourselves what has the power to defy gravity and make life reach skywards. The answer is the sun. It is the heat of the fire element that makes things rise; water to cloud, tree to sky, baby to adult. As the sun pulls life upwards, shadows are cast on the world, their size and shape depending on their angle to the sun.

Felt like the sun was always shining, granting power to be and to act. Also about angles and the shadow warps us, and the size of the shadow is in direct relation to our angle, our relationship to the sun. **If the sun is directly above, there's no shadow**. Like a crocodile.

If you stand with your **back to the sun**, you only see your **shadow**. Crocodiles have their eyes at the back, so they only see the light.

It is a feeling as if I am **dancing with a shadow**.

Dream: **red helium** balloon rising in the distance.

Stand in your truth which is **straight and not crooked**.

The movement into the third dimension seems to involve the use of a tail which can propel living creatures in all three dimensions.

We have lost the **power of tail**, we don't have a tail. It's only our sperm which have tails now. What a tail gives us is extra balance, propulsion and protection.

The letter 'a' is just an 'o' with a tail, which felt wonderful. The capital 'A' is all about support, and it's fine when the H is **upright as it doesn't go horizontal**. The 'A' **horizontally** felt like the open mouth of a crocodile, with a stick in it to keep it open. It felt like I was open from the front.

Here is the symptom in picture form:

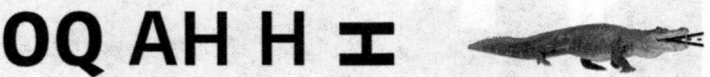

Figure 11.17 Proving symptom in picture form

Finally, the third dimension unfolds in all its glory.

It felt like the time and size were now accurate.

How will it affect the way we feel, behave and live in the world?

Human aspects of the third dimension

With each extra dimension that we acquire, we both lose and gain something. Helium is most free as it is not confined to a body, yet it is also the most restricted because of its linear existence. Neon gains free will but is confined by its two-dimensional desires and aversions. Neon's surface-bound newborn depicts the early development of self, a two-dimensional ego ruled by desire.

Dream the baby is strapped on to the table.

The third dimension rounds out our character and lends depth to our personality. As we grow from crawling baby to upright youth, we enter a new emotional dimension, ready to face the world and form relationships with others. However, concurrent with the development of our light side, we begin to develop a shadow. Shadows are not possible in the flatlands of Neon. To earn our shadow, we must stand upright.

It is true that the shadow is mentioned in Neon as well. This however was a simple back-front, yin-yang division, the flat world of desires and aversions. The full human shadow in its developed form is concealed below the belt. Here hide the urinary, fecal and sexual organs, whose emotional connotations are reflected in the dreams, sexual fantasies and swear words they generate. This tendency begins to develop in early childhood, when a toddler utters his first '*You are a pooh-pooh*' sentence.

By the time we reach puberty we create four variations of light and shade. A front side to show the world, a back to turn to the world, a bottom which is semi-hidden and our sexual organs reserved for those special moments (Figure 11.18). Another way to describe these aspects of self would be superego-façade, ego-hidden thoughts, id-basic animal instinct and sexuality. In terms of our emotional ecology, we now have sun, cloud, earth and root.

We are afraid of our own shadows. Light in nest, mother's body shadows and protects.

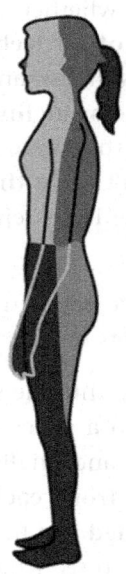

Figure 11.18 *Four degrees of shade*

The pathology of Argon lies in an incomplete or unassimilated form of the shadow, which will reflect in inability to form relationships or to deal with more complex emotional issues, as demonstrated in Chapter 7 Argon 1M Higher emotional themes. This may lead to discontent, grief, irritability, panic attacks and unhappy relationships. Here is one example:

Chaos. I don't know how to be a father. I don't have time to be a mother and still there is no space or time for my work. I feel alone and apprehensive.

How can I create light and beauty and harmony when I am overpowered by disruption?

I am not sure how I am in relationships. Am I safer for others if I am on my own?

An examination of the mental, emotional and spiritual reflections of the third dimension in the proving reveals that as height and depth develop so do more profound emotions. The following is an attempt to come to grips with this new dimension developing deep inside.

Felt good that could spend **days in the sun** and nights in **depths of emotions**.

It was like a wheel being moved by water. Things were being **undermined** and it felt like people were making allegations. '**Undergo**' was how it felt. Not to underestimate and whether to move **below and then above?** It felt like only seeing the **tip of an iceberg and not below**. From the outside is the appearance of stillness and inside there's movement of fullness. You could either **recline or incline**. With the iceberg sensation, it felt like just my eyes, and now they were **above when I was horizontal**, but **when vertical if you didn't have the support of water you could balance on your tail**. It felt like I was rejuvenated, I didn't think I could **flower again**.

We gain the ability to separate between ourselves and others and negotiate the narrow straits of relationships.

The word **intimacy** came up, 'into me see'.

Dream **wedging the car into a space** in an exclusive camping place. People speaking broken French and English. Intense **rivalry**, real **hatred** between two counsellors, **one from each end** of the social spectrum, ending in a huge **lorry overturned** in a field with fire all around it. We are trying to get to the **root of it** – to see whether the driver understands the simple principles involved.

Sensed that the word 'darling' wasn't meant in an **emotional** way, it was just a name to extract information and something you want – it's just a tool.

Along with the depth of emotion, an identity emerges and takes root. As we establish individuality we must test our boundaries against those around us.

Feels like I shouldn't be restricted in any way – **like in society**. Insisting I was right in a situation where I wasn't. Wanting to get my **own way**.

As puberty blossoms we develop sexual characteristics and yearnings. When in harmony these result in loving relationships, but when in the tension of balance, conflict and gender issues arise.

Desire to make love in water.

In the dance, it's only possible at that angle if the **support is mutual**. The dance formed an alliance.

Feeling alive and feminine. Feeling of serenity.

Strong distinction between male and female energy. Female energy is not honoured as it should be. Painful feeling.

All the unconscious impotent rage of the female – suppressed – becomes a vicious self-seeking gossipy, backbiting effort to keep down everyone else as an irrepressible envy fuels all enterprise and thwarts all ambition. First there is volatility, dominance, irritability, anger (a normal state for me) and then the wonderful change comes. The vulnerable heart gives up its old defences.

Eventually emotional maturity evolves, recognising the importance of exploring our shadow side.

Pain can crack the shell, revealing greater understanding. There's a purpose to pain. It's like stalking – like helping the patient stalk themselves to see what's moving, what's dynamic within themselves. Helping them to listen to themselves.

From a mental (intellectual) point of view we must learn to negotiate the three dimensions of space and orientate ourselves correctly so as to perceive reality in the clearest and most accurate way.

Couldn't tell when things were **back to front**, an old symptom from when I was a child – I was always wearing things back to front. When I woke, sometimes I would come into my body the **wrong way around** – either **upside down, back to front** or **sideways on**. I willingly surrender.

I wondered what was different, and the **understanding felt different**. To comprehend fully, to know, to perceive the meaning of. There were lots of explanations that began with 'to'. To catch ideas intended to be conveyed by. To have just and adequate ideas of. To comprehend, to see through. To recognise as implied or meant, although not expressed. To use intellectual faculties to comprehend the power by which one understands. Thinking, reasoning, intelligence **between two persons. Agreements of minds, mutual.** Not to understate the truth. Undertake, to enter upon. Take in hand, to perform.

And like a child growing up we gain the ability to understand complex patterns.

I was understanding letters, numbers and symbols.

Finally, our alignment with the vertical and our expansion into a new dimension brings us one step closer to God. Though we are one step further down the periodic ladder and thus from the source of creation, we are also one step closer to the tenth dimension in which all possibilities happen at once, the return to God.

I didn't have to answer to anyone, only to God. Even when I was disorientated, I was **slipping but correcting** – as though I had an amazing self-correcting mechanism.

In tune with the infinite. The **right angle** in meditation. The angling is also about timing. A **dive with no splash**. Even the water dances. Connected in a mutually supportive way. I am the Way, the Truth and the Light. Only time stalks them.

Feels like before the **serpent lost its legs**. No ego, no separation, just image of God.

Feels like there's just one edge, like of a sword where there's no judgment, no good or bad, no duality. The one edge transforms. The sun rises, I can rest and bask.

The fourth dimension

The three spatial dimensions have unfolded parallel to the three periods, and the third dimension has been completed in Argon. As we descend into the next period the fourth dimension will begin to unfurl. The fourth dimension is commonly considered to be the dimension of time, although there are differing views on this subject. The issue of time is a very prominent one in Krypton. As we have seen previously, there is usually an overlap between adjacent nobles. Argon and Krypton share disorientation as regards to terrestrial time, reflected by these Argon symptoms.

My **time sense** is totally gone. I am frequently 10 minutes late or more – unheard of for me. I have no concept of hours, days, weeks. It could be any amount of time since the proving started. It is as if time didn't exist. I feel that it is completely unmeasured. If it went on much longer I would become terribly frightened because I remember that a sense of time does exist – that this is not real. This could be like madness – or maybe more like **'loopiness'**. Have lost track of days and time since taking remedy.

Disorganised; **late** doing everything.

Delays. Late for things, getting the times of things wrong. Missing connections e.g. trains.

Time was going too quickly for me.

Feeling very rushed for time even though have allowed plenty of it.

The periodic slide – new dimensions

No-thing was every-where
No-thing was every-time.
No-thing was bored.
No-thing decided to pack up its no-things
And go no-where else
But it left some-thing
A dot.

.

Dot was every-thing
Everything was dot.
Dot looked around.
There was no-thing to be seen
Dot tried to move up.
Dot tried to move sideways.
Dot tried to move forward.
It could not. It was dot.
Man, this was frustrating
Dot could not take this for much longer.
Dot got all en-tangled with itself
The pressure was building, fast
Dot was getting mad, real mad
Dot was about to expl-!

Bang.

Dot was free!
It was heaven, it was bliss
One-thing it was not;
Dot became a No-Dot.

Dot expanded
Up, down, back, forward, sideways,
For a million billion whatevers
Dot pushed its own envelope
Expanding into the No-Nothing
Which remained
After No-thing split.

Now No-Dot was Not-Now
And No-Dot was Not-Here
No-Dot had moved somewhere
Between then and there

It rolled and expanded
At incredible pace,
Till Not-Now became time
And Not-Here became space.

But No-dot was scattered
Battered and shattered,
Finding direction
Was all that now mattered.

Because No-Dot was lost
And it looked all around,
No-One to be seen
Not even a sound.

It longed for direction
A place to call home,
And it wished that No-thing
Would pick up the phone.

It wished that No-thing
Would drop it a line,
Just then No-thing called
I hope all is fine?

Here is your line
It's called 'I-me-mine',
Please confine to this line
That leads from up down.

A line? That was fine
I will slide down this line
That extends from mid-heaven
Into some-body's spine.

In a golden shrine
On top of cloud nine,
Line waited its turn
Line bided its time.

Photons forged atoms
Helium fused sun,
Light banished dark
End of day one.

But Line became fixed
Compulsive, Obsessive,
Line would not bend
This got quite excessive.

Dirty or clean
False or be true,
There was really no way
To bridge between two.

Two? You said two?
Knock knock! Two of Who?
Two of two, it is us
And we're saying to you –

Line, Look through the keyhole,
And see what is new,
Break out of your shell
Line, Find the true you.

Set yourself free
I will lend you my strength,
Take a step forward
Break out of length.

More space to play in
Sheet, surface, square,
Combine length and width
There is much power^2 there.

You can tilt to the future
Lean into past,
Scratch till it itches
Reach for the stars.

Well width's what I long for!
Thought Line with a sigh,
I'm tired of floating
Between mud and sky.

I need a good stretch,
He said with a yawn,
I'm bored of this prison
And feeling forlorn.

I needed to flex,
And I wanted to bend,
Time to grow wide now
Time to extend.

Tired of this axis
Heaven and earth,
I'm taking the plunge
I'm going to give birth!

Line took a step forward,
Took a step back,
Opened the door
Heard the shell crack.

Oxygen grasping
Hydrogen's two,
Ozone dividing
Second day through.

Time twisted and curled
Space was a whirl
Universe dancing
Galaxies swirl.

And a star fell from heaven
Split into two,
And he looked at his mom
And he said 'hi what's new?'

Now a baby's a baby
Until it grows ripe,
It functions quite simply
It works like a pipe;

You pump food in one side
Some love and a drink,
And it comes out the other
With quite a big stink

It cries and demands,
It screams till it gets,
It doesn't see others
It doesn't care yet.

There're some babies I know
That at age forty-two
Can't get satisfaction
And scream till they're blue.

So to reach for the stars
Or melt into bliss,
They shoot up some junk
Or just take the piss.

It's a shallow existence
Of joy, discontent,
So we're longing for depth
To give us a vent.

As we float in our ark
Side by side, two by two,
It's time that we turned
And recognised you.

We'll send out a dove,
Open our throat,
Find some expression,
Get off this old boat.

Find us some earth
Let waters recede,
Search for some soil
In which to plant seed.

Earth will grow grasses,
Earth will sprout trees,
Play in the garden
Happy and free.

It was Time to gain height,
It was Time to gain depth,
Take a step sideways
Time to have sex!

And OOOOH Sex felt good,
And OHH Sex felt nice,
No wonder Day Three
Was declared 'it's good' twice!

What makes Sex so special?
The X I am told,
Meiosis crossover
So life can unfold.

But when surface is cubed[3]
From paper to tube,
When flat becomes thick
There's a chance for lovesick.

For a puppy love youth
And a child's Fairy tale,
Can't go on forever
Without getting stale.

When childhood is over
And lovers are gone,
When youth's glow has faded
It's time to move on.

Can't live my whole life
Like an old Peter Pan,
It's time to grow up
To evolve into man.

To be continued . . .

12

ARGON SYNTHESIS

The following is a synthesis of Argon, based on sensations and functions, or the 'verb' of the remedy. Please note that sensation and function are interchangeable and form a cycle.[1] All the expressions below are inseparable and make one totality.

Sensation: Decay
Function: Must preserve.

Sensation: Buried
Function: Must sprout.

Sensation: Two-dimensional ego of a baby
Function: Must grow up.

Sensation: Growing up
Function: Must preserve childhood.

Sensation: Water finds its own level, spread on surface
Functions: Concentrate water to one spot, earth rises to third dimension.

Sensation: Flat
Function: Seek height and depth.

Sensation: Upright with direct connection to heaven.
Function: Forming angles with the sun results in shadows

Sensation: Sun pulling upwards, earth nourishing
Function: Grow tree.

Sensation: Confined by narrow space, obstructed
Function: Create free flow.

Sensation: Connect
Function: Disconnect.

Adjectives:
Yellow, blue, green and red, beautiful, glowing, flowing, obstructed, constricted.

Nouns:
Water, earth, clouds, rain, bog, light bulbs, vegetation, trees upright or felled, passageways, play, dance, grief, depth, basement, attic, baby, teenager, amphibious animals, such as otter and crocodiles, fairies, Peter Pan.

Image:
Preserving blossom to prevent decay.

Vegetation, child and teenager – beauty in full blossom, up-righting and creating new dimensions. But don't ignore the shadow or the roots beneath the earth.

Miasm: Developed Psora. The third period elements are the skin of the earth.

Chakra: Throat

Day of creation: Third

Colour: Blue

Musical scale: G

Whammy: Relationships[2]

Book: Peter Pan

A poem should be palpable and mute
As a globed fruit,

. . .

Silent as the sleeve-worn stone
Of casement ledges where the moss has grown –

. . .

For all the history of grief
An empty doorway and a maple leaf.

For love
The leaning grasses and two lights above the sea –

A poem should not mean
But be.

Archibald MacLeish *Ars Poetica* (1926)[3]

References

1   For more information on this method of synthesis, see Sherr J. *Dynamic Materia Medica – Syphilis: A Study of the Syphilitic Miasm* (2nd edn). Glasgow: Saltire Books, 2015.
2   Sherr J. *The Noble Gases. Helium including an introduction to the Noble Gases.* Glasgow: Saltire Books, 2013.
3   MacLeish A. Ars Poetica. In: *Poetry Magazine*. 1926; **28**(4). Available online at https://tinyurl.com/yb3syw6z

13

ARGON CASES

As well as presenting cases from my practice, and Camilla's, I have collected cases from as many sources as possible to illustrate different aspects of the remedy. The cases are presented in the form in which they were given to me, although they were edited for grammar without changing the meaning.

Some of the follow-ups are long-term and others short. For the purpose of understanding the remedy both are useful. In acute cases the duration of action is naturally shorter.

Note: Expressions relevant to Argon are marked in **bold**

CASE 13.1 Stuck in teens

Jeremy Sherr, Tanzania

Male, 30s

First consultation

Sells spare parts for motorcycles. Loves to ride motorcycles.

Previous homoeopathy: many remedies over several years, none helped.

'My main problem is not wanting to have sex with my wife. Began since she became pregnant four years ago. The idea of sex became strange to me, an alien in her belly, no longer just me and her. After birth, the idea of sex became repulsive, became disgusted at it.

I hate to be pushed into things. I started resenting her for pushing me into this. No logical explanation, she is mad at me, I am mad at her.

I felt innocent, I could not help how I felt.

My sexual desire is normal, this is only with my wife. Before the pregnancy all was well. I keep it secret, an awful thing, can't share it with anyone.

Shy as a teenager, felt not good enough or not good looking enough, no sex as a teenager. My wife was my first sex partner. Difficult in the beginning, took a few days for me to let her get close, for me to let go of the shyness. I wanted to curl up in a ball, **to be loved in an innocent way rather than sexual way.**

I always have an image of **innocent love** instead of sexual love. I was sexual but never in a relationship.

My parents were very loving, good relationship with them. **I was allowed to be a child for a very long time; they never pushed me into being a big boy.** I was allowed to be a kid. As a kid, all was better, no pressure, I could roam the forest and go fishing and do what kids do.

At 15 the girls tried to push me into sex even though I didn't want to. It scared me and I didn't want to be with them. Always longing for beautiful, romantic relationships with the girl of my dreams. My wife was it, just intent, easy to go into sex talk, safe – not physical.

Dark rings around the eyes since 20 years.

I sweat very easily on my back and head, worse with exertion.

Perspiration profuse and offensive, smells like raw meat.

Fungus on feet for 15 years, lately in groin.

Desire for beer and bubbly drinks.

I love to smoke, can't quit.

Lack of energy and easily tired. Very much worse for any mental exertion.

Easily angry, must always suppress my anger or will do something awful. My first feeling is anger, which I suppress.

I hate being pushed into things. Hate and sadness are my main feelings, the only ones I can define.

Injustice or unfairness aggravates. If things don't go my way I get frustrated or angry. I hate stupid people, judgmental. Ignorant people that don't want to be educated. I don't like them therefore I hate them. Either I love people or hate people to hell.

Everyone wants a piece of me. My wife, my son, my clients, all want something from me. Not enough hours in the day to cope with everyone's requests, no time for me to do what I like and want to do. I like motorbikes and working in the garden. But I have to do the things for the house, if I don't do it, no one else will – responsibility.

Difficult to define my role in the family, father, husband or me, can only do one at a time.

Perfectionist, everything must be perfect. I can't stand criticism. Everything must be lined up. Things must be flat. Fastidious, hate mess.

If things don't go smoothly, if it goes difficult, I get mad at the customers. What the fuck do you ask me questions for?

Worked hard in school and did well. I wanted to do art and crafts, but my father talked me out of it and convinced me to be an engineer. I did it to please him.

I can't deal with emotional problems, can't describe my emotions.

Desire to be alone.

Slow at making decisions, irresolute.

I feel like a failure, failure in my relationship. Failure at work. I am highly educated yet I sell oil filters for bikes. Maybe people think I'm stupid. I can't handle responsibilities, can't do work with high responsibility like an engineer. Get stressed from responsibility. Feel too responsible for family. Sense of failure, unhealthy living, beer, smoking, no exercise.

My father was too strict. I wasn't allowed to cry as a kid. Not allowed to contradict him. I piled up anger and negativity all my life. I had both freedom from loving parents as well as restrictions from father.

Dreams of **flying, running fast, longer steps**, can jump up with feet first and fly.

Desire very spicy foods and salt'.

Comment (JS)

Although I felt I understood the issues well, I could not come up with a remedy that fitted the heart of the matter. His issue was an over-extended childhood, which resulted in an innocent and naive state with inability to develop the complex emotional realm of relationships and sexuality. His emotions were simplistic and two-dimensional, either love or hate. The problem exacerbated when his wife became pregnant, like a child who feels rejected during his mother's pregnancy. He could not deal with the multiple roles of father, husband and responsible provider. At the time I did not understand Argon well enough. Instead I concentrated on the other aspects of the case, the perfectionism, frustration and suppressed anger resulting from too strict a father.

Over six months I prescribed Carcinosin and Lac humanum, as well as Carbo vegetabilis and Hepar sulph for acute situations.

There was a good improvement from all the remedies. He became much better with regard to anger, moods, energy, ability to deal with responsibility and stress. He could handle issues much better. Less sense of failure and less overwhelmed. Perspiration and dark circles under eyes improved. Exercising more and feeling good.

But there was no change at all in the main problem – his sexual relationship with wife. I knew I was not hitting the spot.

Follow-up ten months after first visit

'Many things are better but the sexual issue is getting me down.

I am missing my motorcycle brotherhood, lonely.

I miss age 16–18, late teens, I was not ready to be an adult. Sad and cried over it. I wasn't ready for adult life, I was deserted. Sadness became anger, I closed inwards and dwelt in sadness and anger which I cannot express. I wasn't ready to be a father'.

I spoke to his wife: 'The remedies have all helped, less irritable and stressed, more energy, but the main issue remains.

He keeps on going on about being the one who takes care of every-thing. This is how he feels, like there is no one else to take care of things. Caring for the house, car, and our son seems to be too much on top of being at work all the time. **All these jobs that the man of the house needs to do are too much for him.**

He says that things pile up, there are many things that need atten-tion right now and that exhausts him. He **gets stuck with things**.

He cannot ask for help or anything. I think that he needs therapy. I think just remedies won't do it. I am having trouble not getting extremely mad with this victim attitude of 'there is no one else'. **He has to be the hero**, which makes him feel better.

He feels insignificant and useless. He puts all the effort into work so that there is no energy left for anything else, especially not for any-thing that requires emotions, closeness and sex. Talking about it is a no-no because it stresses him. It is hard for me to deal with that. Aversion to company and touch. He is extremely tidy and must line everything up.

He is always reading hero books (Jack Reacher). He reads the same books over and over. Reacher is the man he would like to be. Travel wherever you want and be whatever you want to be, a hero'.

Rx: Argon 200C

Comment (JS)
It was Jack Reacher that triggered the thought of Argon in me. Reacher is a very powerful and noble hero, perfect in every way. He solves crimes, beats up bad guys and beds one woman in each book, but he never needs anyone's company, never sticks around and never forms any lasting relationship. The books are very two-dimensional and repetitive, always following the same pattern, a closed loop. While many people love to read these books, it would be highly unusual to read them twice and more times. (See 'Eye of Argon' in Chapter 16.)

Another important factor in this case is the dreams: Dreams of flying, running fast, longer steps, and flying. These indicate the verb of Argon, the ability to flow, in contrast to his stuck life.

Follow-up one month later
'I had a big aggravation for one week, which is now better.

Severe haemorrhoids, did not want to talk to anyone, just read Reacher. Complete disconnection, all the usual stuff but much worse, did not want any connection and felt horrible. Irritable, just wanted to be left alone and in peace.

After one week I started feeling like being with other people, because I felt lonely. Warm, tender feelings towards my wife and son started appearing. I was missing my family a lot while they were gone. Wanted to do things for the right reason (family) instead of "having to do everything myself". I wanted to be with the family. Happy to deal with people at work. Less cravings for salt and beer, less smoking, less worrying about the house, car, money etc. Started going to bed earlier, falling asleep easier, sleeping deeper. Feeling better mentally. Sweating less, exercising more, lost weight'.

Now he is more communicative and open. His wife is pregnant and he is much more open to it, not horrified like the first time.

His wife writes: 'Since the remedy he has been normal towards me. He looks at me, smiles, kisses me, touches me, and our sex life is back to what it was before our son was born. This has continued the same way even now I am pregnant and my belly is already showing.

His erections are also more powerful and he has been able to have sex in the evenings, which was not possible before. He needed to have slept and be well-rested for that.

His alcohol consumption has also diminished.

He has been sending me "love messages" again'.

His improvement has continued.

CASE 13.2 Caught between past disappointments and uncertain plans for the future

David Johnson, USA

Female, age 42

First consultation
'I've been struggling with depression since March. **My partner left; he moved on.** I can't break out of these old feelings. **I want to have my old life back,** or have a new life. I'm working so hard at just maintaining . . .

I want help getting back in balance. I want to get unstuck.

I had a vision of what my life was going to be. Now that's all changed. I thought I'd grow old with J. We talked about opening a bed and breakfast (hotel). We had a lot of rituals we'd built in over the past eleven years – now that's all gone.

It's hard to re-write my script. It feels like the end for me. I felt terror; **I couldn't breathe.** I felt terror, anxiety, fear. **I just cry for no reason, I break down into tears.** I can't get a grip. I have to go off and hide.

I can't be an emotional wreck at work. Everything's fallen apart. **I'm treading water** but barely maintaining. It shouldn't be this hard. It feels horrible. I don't even know if it's possible to re-write the script'.

Practitioner: Can you describe more about the feelings?

'Loneliness, rejection, replaced, unworthy, not good enough, I'll never be good enough, desperate, pathetic, unlovable, undesirable, disappointed, disillusioned, not trusting, hopeless, exhausted, I can't keep working on this, it's too hard. I feel detached and ungrounded. **Part of me feels like I wasted my youth. I'm old. I'll never find another partner.** I could've found someone to share my life with. I thought that person would be J, but I feel deceived, as if my spirit's crushed. I feel broken.

The relationship is gone. I fought for it and lost the battle. I really wanted another child, but held off because J didn't want to. Now it's too late.

It feels like it's over, almost impossible to start again. It's too late. I've done everything great that I'm going to do in my life: being a mother of two kids was the greatest thing I've done. That's over. Then, I get dumped by my partner. That's over, too.

I'm definitely feeling ungrounded.

I want to escape, but I don't know how or where. I just keep crying and crying.

I can't re-write the old chapter, and don't even know if it's possible to re-write the new chapter'.

Practitioner: More about the feelings?

'I'm stuck in the muck, ungrounded, detached, wanting to escape into my own world. I'm deeply disappointed, I've lost trust, I'm deeply disillusioned with people and their potential. There's loneliness.

I wanted to grow old with someone. I **don't think that will ever happen again. I feel like we were a family, and now we're not. I** felt like we'd grow old together, until one of us died in the other's arms. It's dangerous and toxic for me to hold on to what's gone'.

Practitioner: Can you describe more about "re-writing the script"?

'I used to know what that script was, but now I don't. There's an element of fear. J was a very stabilizing force in my life. It's as if someone pulled the rug out from under me and I don't know how to get that back.

Before I met J I had chronic fatigue syndrome. I was sick for many years. I was really lonely. My whole sense of the universe was shaken. It was a frightening, frightening, lonely journey – **very disconnected**.

I'd see couples all around me. I'd wish I had a partner who was there day to day, who would be present, supportive, there for me, someone to be there for me. It was a feeling of total isolation. I felt **cut off from everyone, completely alone**, really afraid, like I was dying'.

Practitioner: Any tendencies to sense other people's energies?

'Yes, all the time. I can feel what's going on with them even before they tell me'.

Practitioner: Dreams?

'I have a recurrent dream of driving in a car. I come to a crossroad, with the unknown up ahead. **I always decide to go back into the familiar. I'm afraid of moving forward. There's a fear I'll be lost, not ever reaching a final destination.** It's like I want to move forward. It looks magical, mystical, but I'm seized by fear and I have to go back to what's familiar. The stability along with the unknown creates a sense of excitement. **There really could be something beyond'**!

Assessment

The client describes an extreme state of sadness and disconnection, not able to leave thoughts of the past, nor able to move forward into a new life. She feels ungrounded. Although she feels disconnected, she also has the ability to sense others' energies.

The noble gases, at the far right of the periodic table, are known for a state of dormancy (or 'limbo') – almost like a winter solstice, where one season has ended and another has yet to begin. If the table is drawn in a spiral, then it's easier to see how a noble gas resides between the element preceding it, and the next heavier element following it. In this client's case, she describes a sadness and disappointment of separation, caused by the break-up with her partner, and the feeling that she'll never be able to build another family. So her experience sits between muriaticum (connection/disconnection; sadness, disappointment) and kali (family, structure).

Rx: Argon LM 2

Follow-up two and a half months later
'I'm feeling very good. I just started the LM 3. By two weeks things just turned around for me. I had a turnaround; I've been feeling really good. Everything shifted; it was dramatic.

There was a dream of a threat – these guys were trying to rape me. I had a feeling "I'm going to get out of this", and I did. I woke up feeling liberated. I didn't feel unsettled. It was almost like a triumph.

I've been feeling much more grounded, hopeful, confident, optimistic, connected. My job's really challenging, but not stressing me out. My overall energy is good. It's been better with the remedy, better than it's ever been. Sleep has been good. I'm happy, relieved with the turnaround'.

Rx: Argon LMs The client has continued with new LM remedies about every two months for the past year, keeping in touch as needed (due to financial circumstances she has not followed up directly in the office).

Phone follow-up one year later
'I was doing really well for eight months or so. Things were getting back on track and I was feeling wonderful. Then a series of problems started happening at my job, where I was asked to teach and I have no teaching experience. Then I broke my ankle and I was completely dependent on others. An eleven-month relationship ended at the same time that I broke my ankle – he left me for another woman (laughing).

Even though I experienced a lot of anxiety when all that was happening, the feeling of disconnection wasn't as strong. I came out (recovered) from those experiences much faster than I would have in the past.

When I take the remedy, I feel much less anxiety. It also really helps with my energy levels. I'd like to go up to the next higher potency'!

Rx: Increase to Argon LM 9; continue follow-ups as needed

As this person continues in her healing journey with Argon, she's ever-more resilient and optimistic about moving on with her life. She even laughed (ironically) when relating the story of her latest break-up.

Case first published in Hpathy Ezine, March, 2011

Comment (JS)
Note the reaction to the relationship breakup, which is similar to that of Natrum muriaticum, lots of grief and endless crying. However unlike typical Nat mur relationships, which are often incompatible, in this case the relationship seemed to be perfect, a puppy love that simply went stale. The partner moves on, while she remains stuck in the old dream with a feeling she has wasted her youth. Now she can't breathe, is treading water and feels ungrounded, typical Argon expressions that relate to the first part of the third day of creation, all sea with no ground.

The feeling of a perfect relationship that will be preserved into old age and culminate in a perfect mutual death in each other's arms is typical of Argon. Her dream says it all: *'At a crossroad, with the unknown up ahead. I always decide to go back into the familiar. I'm afraid of moving forward. There's a fear I'll be lost, not ever reaching a final destination. There really could be something beyond'.*

CASE 13.3 Light bulbs
Jeremy Sherr, Tanzania

Female, age 43

First consultation
Previous remedy: Limenitis bredowii California
    Occupation: massage therapist and dancer.
    'I thought I would teach but I can't, it's too big for me. I ran away, felt I am not giving enough. I wanted to give the whole **feeling of motion**, but could not convey it. I can imagine the lesson and the

dance, but when it comes to it I freeze. Maybe the feeling of not good enough, sensitive to opinion of others.

Trying to get pregnant, I left a boyfriend two years ago. Like dance, **not connected to people and society.** I want a boyfriend and family to connect to society. When not working **I disconnect.** I am living in chaos.

I am not really there with boyfriend – only when we separate, I love him. After we separate, the love comes. When in the relationship I become critical, or see the flaws in my partner, or why he doesn't need me.

I am into body language. I imagine people understand my body language, dance or sex, that people could read me that way.

I am nice and full of energy, but turned on or turned off, sit at home and stare.

I would like to be more doing, manifestation not so disconnected.

I like to feel the now, but I don't manifest it. Once I thought all will be ok and things will just happen, maybe I don't see things right, only after a long time.

I like to give all my energy, I have big energy, all seems live and strong and physical, over-confident, over-happy.

As a child I hid behind a tree, would look at people and try to understand how you have to be, how do they do it? **I try to connect to society. Would like to connect to work.** Only connected when dancing, sex.

Easily offended. feeling of being alone, isolation. **Can't flow** with girlfriends.

Lots of anger, but I can't express it, suppress it, keep it in a long time then explode. Huge anger from childhood. I blocked all feelings to mother, no closeness, no hugs.

I was offended and blocked myself off. I always felt she thought others were better, more clever, more beautiful. Lack of confidence and low self-esteem. I don't understand the boundaries and borders.

Desires: carbs, meat, sweet, ice cream, chocolate, fruit

Aversion: seafood, strong smells.

Digestion is sluggish.

Sun aggravates my skin. Photophobia from the sun.

Cold extremities. I like changes in weather, like storms and vol-canoes.

Dream from childhood (you will you laugh at me). A hill, we are playing, two come and put me in the fridge and interrogate me about my parents.

One time I suffered incest abuse, soft rape. I disconnected, left my body, thought I will be ok till I know how to do it. I plan my feelings or think my feelings. Fear of rape.

Third generation holocaust survivor.'

Rx: Germanium 12C, daily for two weeks

Comment (JS)
I missed Argon through not knowing the remedy well at the time. Instead, I focused on the rape, suppressed anger, sensitivity to opinion of others, offended, disconnected and holocaust history. Perhaps she did need Germanium first, to clear out many of her traumas and bring the real picture to the fore.

Follow-up two months later
'After the remedy I felt very good, much better, not floating. Felt light, slept better.

Met a man and fell in love and had a relationship.

Generally, much better all round.

I am a new person. Left my old work, looking for new directions. Amazing! I can't believe it'.

Rx: Germanium 12C, daily for two weeks

Follow-up two months later
'Gone back a bit.

Big plans or tiny plans. Don't realise my plans, I wait.

Been waiting for years for a baby but didn't wake up that time was passing. I am now 43. I was going to go to the sperm bank so many times but just didn't do it. Waiting for sperm, hope it's not too late.

Cracked lips.

I make plans but nothing happens.

Much better than before, all original symptoms gone.

Dreams of marriage. Waiting for years to get pregnant, now, at 43, not doing anything about it, just make plans and they don't happen.

Dream of a wedding. I am in a bar, a blonde woman says, "Look, that guy made me drunk, I won't marry him". Then I am in a house on the second floor, the bride and the groom are going to jump, each in his turn, with a rope. She is very scared. When she jumps, it goes wrong. I try to catch her and can't and she falls. I run down with the rope. I go back up, lots of girls whispering, an older, naked woman is there.

Dream of a wedding, renting a room, wedding hall, people not my style, they give me an ugly ring. It is a wedding so I marry their son, my parents are there. I say, "Oh well, this is not really happening". After the party we go out with the ring and groom, then I say, "You know I can't kiss you". But then I realise, no, I have to, I am married, this is not a game, I can't walk away, there is a ring, I must be with him even if don't like him. I am in shock, how did I marry and not think of what comes after.

Dream of a hawk diving down and digging dirt from ground that flies in my face.

One more thing, I don't know if this is important. Last week **all the light bulbs burst**, all the phones broke, all electric bulbs blew, the computer broke. This happens all the time, I have many electric issues'.

Rx: Argon 200C

Comment (JS)
While the Germanium was close enough to help it did not hit the spot. The Argon issues of this case, especially the lack of connection and inability to form a relationship are clear, as are the dreams of thwarted or incomplete marriage. As a dance teacher she seeks to move, but is inert and cannot manifest anything. In her first dream she is preserved in a fridge. Interesting extra points are, waiting for sperm and the up-down dimension that appears in the dream, as well as the ground flying in her face. Her expression in the first case, of being turned on and off, resonates with her electric problems.

Follow-up six weeks later
'I feel so great, amazing!!
   I have never felt so good.
   I had a romance, everything is light and smooth. All goes well.

No indecision, no anxiety, just loads of energy and strength, I have felt so good, wonderful! As if someone took the heaviness out of me that I carried all my life.

Had three dreams of murder or killing and something flies away from me and I wake feeling really good. Or dream someone has killed people and wants to escape, then I feel I can catch or understand something I didn't understand before.

I feel so good maybe I should not be allowed to feel this good!

Things are flowing much better in my life.

I am eager to meet someone now, very open to a relationship. This is new – the ability to be with the right person.

Wow, I want to eat the world'!

Rx: Nil

Improvement continues.

CASE 13.4 Alone with camera, crushed into 2D

Charlotta Åström-Lynch Helsinki, Finland

Male, age 40

First consultation

He is from Southern Europe, but has lived abroad for two decades. He makes **animation films** for a living. He has had awful nightmares ever since he was a little kid.

He also has skin problems and suffers from restless legs. The skin rash is desquamating, behind the ears, on the eyebrows and on the chest. Some itchiness, worse from stress.

'I feel very stressed. My girlfriend got pregnant but **I never wanted kids**. I always made that clear to everyone. She really wanted a baby for the last few years, she got depressed. Now that she is pregnant I got depressed. **I don't know how to deal with it.** Since then stress and nightmares are much worse. It's not a very nice situation, **like in a limbo**. I want to get it right. My mind is the trouble.

I am an independent, closed person. **I have my own world. I find it hard to relate.** I have always lived on my own. Moving in together was a big step, very difficult at the beginning. **This pregnancy is another step I'm really scared of. I don't normally open up.** This is the next big step'.

(He visited a homoeopath 3 years ago with nightmares and restless legs; he got Mercurius.)

Practitioner: Tell me about the stress?

'I take my work seriously. I really like to do it. I work very hard, and become stressed if it's not going well. The nervousness piles up, I get anxious, I get nightmares. I get stressed over deadlines, I push myself all the time. I am thinking about it all the time'.

Observation: he shows chaotic motion of hands and he is frequently squeezing his head with his hands.

He is a skilled photographer; this hobby is almost an obsession. He takes photos, mostly of people. Loves travelling and photographing normal people, interesting people.

'I am very shy, **kind of closed.** It is a kind of one-to-one shyness; it is easier to be open in a group. It's a sort of fear of people, I am not sociable, used to be more but now less and less. I was extremely shy as a kid. Wouldn't speak, wouldn't get out of the car. It was a nightmare to meet new people, distant relatives, parents' friends. Scared, horrible experience. **Most of the time I spent in the car, reading comics. I love graphic novels.**

School was different. I was OK there, even outgoing.

Our family were never very close. Never spoke much to each other. Parents were conservative, very religious. I always had many friends though! I became a rebel, studied photography, went abroad. I always looked up to my uncle and auntie, they had no kids, they used to travel a lot. I didn't want my parents' life, all work, struggling, difficult. My uncle and auntie were free'.

Practitioner: Tell me about the nightmares.

'I have had them since I was 3 years old. As a teenager I used to wake up screaming. But they were unremembered.

Very violent. Falling down some cliff, I would get out of bed and try to cling onto something. Travelling in a car very fast, trying to stop.

Snowboarding down a slope.

Going under something and getting crushed. On a boat going very fast, **smashing into something. Ceiling falling down on me and I get squashed.**

I am half asleep, half awake, my eyes are open – I see someone in the room, a stranger. It takes a while to realize it's a nightmare and not real.

They come and go. Some weeks I have the same nightmare all the time.

Sometimes they come straight after falling asleep. Sometimes, I open my eyes – see the curtain, and it becomes part of the nightmare. Some object in the room can trigger it. I can be awake – and yet see something. It never happens in the daytime. I will scream in my native language, sometimes I will start getting dressed.

The nightmares are worse if I eat late in evening.

Often I don't even remember what has happened afterwards, but my girlfriend tells me.

I take quite a while to fall asleep. Thinking, thinking, thinking. Nightmares are worse during periods when my brain is very active. I have always had a very active mind. It's all stuff I'm working on, making the whole thing in my head'.

He has had no violent experiences in the past.

Birth was normal, but as a baby used to cry and cry, non-stop. Had acne in puberty into 20's, worse on forehead.

Very hot, easy perspiration of torso. Not during the dreams, however. Feels worse in hot weather.

Restless legs all day long and when in bed, feels electric, worse when moving the legs. At work will constantly shake one leg and also in the evening when on the sofa.

'I'm quite impulsive, irritable. I react disproportionately, I snap at people. Hard to keep up conversation. I don't have any patience. I **feel blocked.** Not relevant, not of interest. Nobody really knows me. I feel at my best alone with my camera somewhere'.

Scoliosis.

Allergy to pollen, dust, cats.

As a teenager, had epistaxis in the spring.

Eats everything, dislikes spices. A very strong **desire for plain yoghurt**, he eats litres per week for breakfast, lunch & dinner, plain or with fruits and cereals. Aversion plain milk, swede, water chestnuts. Thirstless.

Rx: Argon 1M split dose, then 30C once weekly

Assessment
The aversion to marriage, desire for freedom, expansiveness, hot constitution and skin problems brought to mind the gaseous neighbors of Sulphur – Oxygen, Nitrogen, Chlorum and Fluor. However, there was something about the isolation, the speed of his mind, the 'superheroness' of his work, mind and dreams that made me think he needed a noble gas. I chose the third period partly because the skin symptoms reminded me of Sulphur, but even more so because the third period, according to Andreas Bjørndal's work on the periodic table, is to do with relationship and communication issues. Noble gas, third period – Argon. I had no previous knowledge or experience of this remedy.

Follow-up
He has had one single nightmare during this period, it came the first night after the 1M. He was going down a waterfall, at a high speed.

Since then no nightmares, no other lucid states at night.

After the first three doses, he got very depressed but then got better within a few days. One week later, got depressed just the day before the next dose of 30C, after which the following morning felt light, like a black cloud had lifted.

No more dips into depression after that.

The skin or the scalp got really dry for the past 4 weeks, getting better now.

Restless legs are still there.

More ok with the baby, started telling his family about it.

Stress levels at work are high, deadlines coming up. That makes him restless, waking up at night. An electric feeling in the body. Always gets stressed around deadlines.

Feeling better around people, but still annoyed by their loudness.

Feeling a bit more positive.

Still gets thinking a lot before falling asleep, but not too bad!

Desire yoghurt – still the same amount, 4 litres a week. Aversion, plain milk. Not even as a child on the farm. Aversion goat's milk. Desire cheese.

Started sneezing last weekend (pollen allergy). This usually comes more towards the summer.

The back has been quite alright.

Rx: Argon 30C, drops as required

Follow-up three months later
'Feeling quite ok since the last time.
 But in the past 2 weeks nightmares returned, every night now.
 No amelioration from the 30C'.
 He has taken 3 doses of 30C this summer.
 'Nightmares have been different this time, more violent.
 Girlfriend wakes me, takes a long time. Now I've started shaking her (before wasn't aware of her at all in the dreams).
 Mostly it's the window or the curtains turning into the nightmare, I am trying to escape.
 Like a huge door. Like being in between – an open door and something to do with outside the room.
 It's a door or window and light. I also had a weird experience, I was sitting in a room and it felt as if spiders were spinning a web around me. I am talking a lot in the dream with my girlfriend.
 The dreams no longer involve smashing/speed'.
 This relapse was after he came back from a trip abroad and was just about to go back to work. Stressed by work, waking up stressed in the mornings with a tense jaw and tense muscles.
 'Not happy to come back to work. The language isolates me a lot. I like the work, but not the company. I'm the only foreigner. Don't like the people, they are robotic. You never know what they think. They never tell you straight to your face.
 The pregnancy is now 6 months, more relaxed about it'.
 If he gets depression, just a few drops of the remedy has helped.
 Physical health has been good. Still a lot of restless legs.
 Since he went back to work, back pain and the skin is worse again, desquamation, oily stuff.

Rx: Argon 1M, split dose, which again brought about significant improvement

He has remained well. He has a baby now and still repeats Argon in the 1M potency from time to time. So far, the remedy still improves his condition when repeated.

Comment (JS)
This case has several similarities to Case 1 in terms of the childish inability to grow up and the inability to deal with his partner's pregnancy. It is interesting to note the dreams of traveling at speed but being obstructed or smashing into things, and of the ceiling falling on him. These represent his inability to move from the second dimension to the third dimension. Likewise, he sees the world through flat 2D photographs. After the remedy, a door opens wide, and he can fall down the waterfall into the third dimension of height, and with it acquire the ability to relate to others. Note also the desire for plain yogurt – baby food. The Argon theme of boats is also present.

CASE 13.5 Between a serious person and a freedom-loving person

Jeremy Sherr, Tanzania

Male, age 35

First consultation
Young man, smiley, a nice twinkle.
   He found out he had a melanoma so he went into industrial cannabis cultivation, growing cannabis commercially for health industry.
   He has had homoeopathy before but only for acutes.
   'I like working outside and with nature; it's open and it's an escape. I'm a sensitive person. Sensitive to many things.
   Should I go on as a worker or do something commercial, between individual worker and commercial? On the cusp, between a serious person and a freedom-loving person. I wonder if I should take responsibility and decisions; I used to avoid it.
   Haemorrhoids for six months and a fissure.
   Many operations, nothing big, a torn ear drum, compartment syndrome from a broken ankle.
   I dehydrate easily. I have a constant lack of fluid.
   Things happen in twos, left and right, symmetrical, semi. Half-symmetrical, happen in twos – two ears, two melanomas.

Not fulfilling myself in work. A gap between me and other workers'.

Observation: He is airy, theoretical, higher consciousness, sensitive, idealist "new-agey".

'I am a thinker, more of an idealist than a commercial worker in the cannabis industry.

With me it is very clear, **I feel that I am lying to myself**. Living a life of not doing 100%, not doing the things you really believe in. The lying is being with **people that are not 100%** and that are not serious.

There is a gap between me and the day workers – they are not committed.

I am looking for freedom and business combined; looking to combine both in a wholesome way.

I am **disconnected from family and old friends**; that doesn't bother me, but it bothers them.

It feels whole to me, adventure and anonymity.

A gap between me and them, not normal contact.

There is a gap (same as with the workers).

The old friends are into lad things and I am different. If I need to meet them it takes my time, and I **like to be alone**, don't want to divide my time with a social life; I want to be anonymous.

I feel comfortable alone'.

Observation: There is a gap between his round and wholeness, and their imperfections.

'**My old world had less responsibility, more freedom in my head**, more sociability, more girls.

Now I try to do things in a **wholesome way**.

It needs a lot of responsibility to grow the grass. I am the lowest in the system but take most of the responsibility; that is the gap.

In the army I didn't tell people lots of things, I kept them to myself. Not necessarily tell the truth.

I need to **keep moving**, have to work outside.

But **very calm** too, I can sit and do nothing.

I am most calm and connected, or work 12 hours a day. I am both and I am whole with being both.

I have been dehydrated from a young age for no reason, during travels, headache and vomit. I was sporty, hard and strong but vomited and was dehydrated.

I can drink a lot but it all runs out through perspiration.
I can get sunstroke
I smoke a lot of dope, cannabis calms me.
Vegetarian, like to work with plants.
Desire wholesome food'.

Rx: Argon 200C

Comment (JS)
His main conflict is between a young new-age idealist and the looming grown-up world of commercialism and responsibility. It is difficult for the idealist in him to reconcile with those who do not share his love of truth and of being 100% committed. He seeks to combine both worlds, that of the youthful adventurer and the business-orientated adult, but he remains split between the two. He can be calm and still but must keep moving, and is whole with both. Note the theme of water running out through perspiration leading to dehydration, as well as the love of plants. All are third day issues.

Follow-up two months later
'Much better all round.
   Everything has improved greatly.
   I feel very awake'.
   Observation: He looks much more alert and present.
   'Doing much more, moving ahead.
   I feel Argon is working very well. Both body and mind functioning better.
   Better with people, more positive.
   More alive, more here, no gaps. More connected to here and now.
   Argon gave me the confidence to come out and be my true self.
   I feel I am coming back to life.
   I wanted to tattoo Argon on my arm.
   With the first dose I felt my whole body melt in a gas. I feel like a gas. My skin opened. It brings out my inside, my real self, makes all the fuzziness clear. It retuned me.
   Physically much better too. More awake, joints smoother and better, more athletic, can do more, exercise more. Eating much better.
   Ready to stop drugs now. No more questions, all is clear. I am ready to stop drugs and alcohol.'

Rx: Argon 10M

Follow-up one month later
One month since stopped all drugs.
> Had lots of energy and feels great.
> He left work and is looking for a new direction. Study?
> All hemorrhoids gone, so much better overall.

Rx: Argon 10M

CASE 13.6 Side-tracked

Camilla Sherr, Tanzania and Kate Gathercole, UK

Male, age 26

First consultation
He has a mental disorder and is currently in assisted living accommodation.
> Undiagnosed condition – **possibly a form of autism**. He is accompanied by a support worker.
> Observation: Tall, lean, red-haired, quick to smile and easy laughter, playful, affable.
> 'I'm a little bit **lazy** – I like to sleep. I can't get going, my motivation is low. It's worse in the mornings – I can't get up until after midday.
> I go to bed late – about 1am or later. I listen to the radio and stay up. I don't feel too bad from it – just a little bit tired.
> **I do things slowly.** I wash up slowly – go at my own pace. Other people would like me to speed up a bit.'
> Support worker: It takes you 20 minutes to wash up one mug!!
> '**I like a clean plate.** I take my time – don't rush.
> I feel a bit sluggish. I have problems with my daily routine. The structure to my day is a bit wonky, late nights and late mornings. . . . I'm going at my own pace.'
> Comment: The social workers were worried that he wasn't eating when he lived on his own.
> 'I have trouble saying no, I'm a bit too nice. These kids were preying on me, pestering me, taking my money. There were 5–6 of

them. They were always knocking on the door, pestering me and shouting up at me.

Comment: **He was too nice – he gave in too easily.** Social workers were worried about safety issues.

'Things got tight at home. **Dad pushed me out.** I got help from the social workers – I was attending a day center. I liked playing pool – and gardening.

I had a problem with time then too. I wouldn't get there until the session was nearly finished. I always seem to struggle with it. I get side-tracked. I'm never ready on time. It isn't even the getting ready that's the problem – it's getting started!

It doesn't do my health good, getting up late. I feel sluggish. I feel good in the evening, but it takes me 3 hours to get ready for bed. I'm trying to get back on track.

I get pains in my chest, muscular spasms, Terrible pain.'

Comment: He gets panic attacks with them. He ends up in hospital very frequently.

'I've had scans of my chest, but they can't find anything wrong. The pains in my chest feel like they go high and then burst and come down again. I get breathless with them, constantly blowing out. It feels as if my back is caving in as well. I get pains down my arms and into my shoulders. My arm feels hooked, bowed. They are sharp pains. They're worse if I mow the lawn. It's muscular – like I've strained or pulled something. It feels like I'm having a heart attack.'

Comment: He calls the ambulance all the time. He's been to hospital about 8 times with it.

'With the panic attacks I get spaced out – short of breath, I feel on edge. **I felt like I was flying**, out of control. It's always worse at night when there's no one else around.

I didn't like it in hospital – I felt as if I was picking up germs.

I'm afraid of heights – I get dizzy. I don't have any other fears.

I worry about my mother – her health. I try to be helpful.

I've got a good appetite. I like to eat! I love meat. If it's put in front of me I'll eat it, as long as it's not too hot or spicy.

I get eczema on my hands. I used to get it on my shins.

I'm normally coldish, never hot. I don't like the weather too hot or too cold.

My sleep is very good – too good.

I loved school – I had a good bunch of friends. I looked forward to going.

But it was a big transition at the end of school. I felt like it was all over. Instead of mixing with my friends, I was mixing with adults. I lost contact with people. Everyone was taking different paths. They branched off and we lost contact. It felt like it all had to stop. I had to get on with things.

I'm generally laid back and easy going. **I go with the flow.** I get angry, but I don't get aggressive. I get angry if people pester me. I get angry with myself if I'm not achieving anything.

I'm very laid back'.

Comment: He finds it difficult to say no. He's charming, and unable to say no, he likes to please people.

'It feels as if time goes quickly. **I'd like to wind the clock back a bit'.**

Rx: Argon 200C, single dose

From the Argon proving:

A sense of being suspended in some time zone where movements and actions are slowed down.

Felt time was going too quickly for me, but was not irritated by this, as I would normally be.

Follow-up three weeks later
'Nothing happened.

I can't get out of bed – I need lots of prompting'.

Comment: You don't get so irritated by the prompting though. Things seem a little better.

'I'm still going to bed very late.

I feel slow, sluggish, then once I get going it's ok.

My eczema has been worse – on my shins. It's itchy at the back of my legs. My hands are better but my legs are worse.

I don't really get angry – I get angry with myself if I've done something wrong.

Time goes quick.

My social life is good. I've branched out. Met a few other people.

I saw my mum and dad last week. I saw my brother too. I'm less worried about my mum'.

Comment: His mum said he seemed better when they saw him.

'I went away with my brother – it wasn't too bad. I got myself up ok. I wanted to get on with things – I didn't want to lie around.

I haven't had any chest pains'.

Rx: Wait

Follow-up four weeks later
'I'm picking up a bit, speeding up a bit – I feel I'm getting there.

There's been a little bit of improvement.

I feel more confident – more assertive.

Time has gone quick since our last appointment.

I've been doing normal things. Went to my parents at Easter – it was real good.

I went out with some friends last week – I stayed awake all day and all night.

The eczema is still bad. It feels hot and itchy. It's ok if I don't think about it. It's nice to scratch!

Everything's been smooth'.

Comment: He's taking less time washing up – only a few minutes on each cup. There are times when he gets up ok. We noticed a change – it's getting a lot easier. Much better.

'I've no worries – not worried about my mum.

No problems with the chest.

I had a funny dream – I was running late and they were pushing me to get going'.

Social worker: He has been much more confident and assertive – up front, **confronting things that are bothering him.**

'My social life could be better – I'm trying to hook up with people.

Mealtimes are still a little out of sync. **I still get a bit side-tracked.**

I still feel a bit sluggish, but not so lethargic – **now I'm flying'.**

Rx: Wait

Follow-up four weeks later
'Eczema is still bad on the right shin, a bit scabby. The skin feels tight and itchy. Left leg is better now. I need to balance up.

Still, a big improvement getting up in the morning'.

Comment: He's very assertive – had a few run-ins with other house members.

'**I made a flying visit to my parents – flew through the door –** it was a flying visit. I was a bit late.

Time just goes like that. It goes quick. I'd love to turn the clock back a bit. I'm not utilising time correctly. I can't keep up with time and things that are going on'.

Rx: Argon 1M

Follow-up six weeks later

'I dropped towards the end of last week. My chest came over a bit light – I felt very light.

I'm working at the minute. Picking up a few things. I need to improve – need to be an asset. Not look like a bloody idiot.

My leg was itchy yesterday and this morning – it hasn't been too bad.

I get easily side-tracked.

I go to bed late and get up late . . . playing catch-up all the time'.

Comment: There hasn't been so much improvement in the past month. . . . If anything he's gone backwards.

Rx: Argon LM4

Follow-up six weeks later

'I've had more good days, doing very well.

I'm working – plumbing and heating. I have ups and downs with it – but it is good experience. I'm getting there ok.

I had some pains in the chest, when I was in bed. Sort of spasms. They got better again by themselves. Lasted maybe an hour.'

Social worker: He coped with them really well – he didn't get so anxious about them . . . not like he used to – he always used to call out the ambulance.

'Eczema is ok – no itching'.

Generally doing very well.

Rx: Continue Argon LM4

Comment (JS)

This young man reminded Camilla of Peter Pan, always talking of flying. He was stuck in time, both in terms of inability to grow up and leave home and school and being unable to move forward in time on a daily basis. He is always side-tracked and late. After the remedy, time seems to speed up, allowing him to move on. In his dreams he is late but is now being pushed to get going. He becomes less childlike and defenseless and is able to confront people and problems. Everything flows better and seems smoother, a new dimension has opened up and he is flying.

CASE 13.7 Follows Natrum muriaticum

Jeremy Sherr, Tanzania

Female, 30s

This is a young woman I have seen sporadically over a few years. She did quite well on Thuja and Positronium, but I had not seen her for quite some time until she returned for this consultation.

'I have career issues, fighting for position in a job. An aggressive component, strong goals and I will make them happen. People judge me for not doing things the right way and I get offended'.

Nausea worse for heartbreak. Once again, she was left broken-hearted.

Dream of people she quarreled with apologising to her. Sense of injustice. 'People make me feel I'm not doing a good job and I lose confidence'.

Warts on finger.

Desire acid and vinegar.

Connected to animals.

Secretive, can't be out in the open with relationships. Main problem is relationships. 'I always pick non-available men'.

Rx: Natrum muriaticum 1M

Follow-up two months later
'Much better, felt very good on Natrum muriaticum'.

Rx: Natrum muriaticum 10M, when needed

I then did not see her for 20 months.

Follow-up 20 months later
'I feel ugly and unlovable. I want to not be so hard on myself, then I could find a partner. I want a romantic relationship'.
   Dream of long journeys and being locked out of places.
   Right-sided problems.
   'Either I have collapse and exhaustion, **don't want to move, or I go fast, fast, fast,** no one fast enough. Eagle eyes – sharp, incisive, see things clearly. Fast, impatient and do a lot of things. Then catatonic, all heavy and slow **can't move like walking in molasses.**
   Acne eruptions-make me feel ugly. Symmetrical.
   Desire acid, vinegar, ice cream.
   Warts on fingers.
   Severe itching on legs.
   Dream of a complex building, many levels going down, further and further. Dream of a journey, leading a group of people, **feel lost but I carry on, with trials and difficulty that doesn't let me get to the goal.**
   Romantic – but attracted to people not available. Not believing I am enough, unattractive feeling, **but sometimes feel beautiful'.**

Rx: Argon 200C

Comment (JS)
As we will see, Argon has a strong similarity and relationship to Natrum muriaticum. Both remedies may be broken-hearted, but there are some themes that indicate Argon. The patient is youthful but has always had problems with relationships, confidence and self-esteem, yet at times she feels beautiful. The acne and its emotional connotation is also a teenage sign. The theme of obstruction and free flow is apparent in her life and the dreams.

Follow-up two months later
'Fantastic remedy!
   Definitely helped me, made me very happy.

Big spurt of energy, lots of organizing and clearing out. All seemed clearer, I could **move through things faster and much less stuck-ness**.

Itchy legs much better, huge relief.

Less ugly and unlovable. Less hard on self.

Easier to do things, much less exhaustion.

Acne better. Warts better.

Dream of murdering someone, (my boss). I was very angry with him.

Change with the romantic feeling, I am being noticed more and respond better.

Rx: Argon 200C, when needed

Follow-up three months later

She feels much calmer and better. Left job and started own business.

'Working less hard. Don't feel I have to earn my keep so much, OK just to be me. Working for myself, much better.

Repeated remedy two times, felt better every time.

Cleaned house a lot. A psychic and physical cleaning.

Forgiving mother after many years, not holding on to anger.

Some eczema on fingers itchy, now clearing up.

Fantastic remedy, huge step forward'.

Rx: Argon 200C, when needed

CASE 13.8 French Mistress

Sara Kabariti, Jordan

This is the account of a patient after receiving a dose of Argon 200C. The remedy helped her in several ways, but was not fully curative and a partial proving occurred. As the patient is very sensitive and expressive, she paints an interesting impression of Argon.

Observation: Patient is wearing a pink, light fuchsia, almost fluorescent top. She was wearing a similar coloured top yesterday too! **Looks like a teenager.**

'The remedy is like the mistress of a French man. She's not old, but she's older than a teenager and the feeling is of a **lull in time**. Like when you take your first sip of white wine on an empty stomach. It's yellow, it's light, it's a flower (by the way, yellow isn't my colour). It's floral, like freesia almost.

The sense of smell is very strong with this remedy. I smell everything subtle or heavy. If it attacks a sense, it's the sense of smell.

The perspective turns. I started to look at things more lightly. It's not intense. The reason I can feel it a lot is because it's exactly the opposite of what I am. It's always in a grey area, there's nothing black or white, right or wrong, it's all swimming in the grey. Nothing seems very important; not in a detached way but because I'm so carefree.

This remedy has a bit of selfishness to it, like a mistress. The mistress isn't as intense as the wife because everything is taken care of, **all is provided with no responsibility.**

I tell you why I know this, because I'm rereading Herman Hesse's *The Glass Bead Game*. I had to put that down because the intensity just isn't there. So I pick up a book for my book club; *Only in London*; all about sluts.

This remedy makes one quite selfish like a mistress. The wife sacrifices and is there; the mistress is there **but in the end all is for her benefit.**

This remedy is all woman, very attractive. I'm lazing around; like the French mistress, not like a Bangkok hooker. She's all woman but she's silent, strong, she knows a lot but doesn't tire herself. Almost like a feline reclining. Makes you so horny; a lot. All I want to do is lie in bed.

I got my period on Tuesday. It's a little bit different – usually it's very heavy. This time it barely stained the pad but a lot comes down with the urine. As if it has something to do with gravity. With urine, as if it propels it more. Why am I using the word propelled? Never used it in my life.

For me, the thread is like observing in a very relaxed way. It doesn't make you feel rushed. For me, nothing has changed in my busy schedule but I seem to be more at ease.

If I wanted to describe this remedy – it rounds off sharp edges. Nothing is sharp'.

Practitioner: Has it helped you?

'This is carefree but it has no depth. I can't imagine living like this forever. This is a holiday remedy. Good for somebody in a situation they can't get out of right now.

Like a first aid remedy, I would say, because it softens; there's no intensity, nothing seems so bad. Like taking a break from the real deal. It's a bit frivolous, superficial, light, non-threatening; a French mistress but one who's well taken care of. French, because in their culture, they expect a man to have a mistress, so there are no morality issues going on. No deep thoughts.

It's material in a way. Today in yoga, of all places, I am thinking I need to buy a gold ring. But not extravagant – there's a dress-up element to it.

It's like I'm just hanging out, enjoying. Spring, but it's dainty growth. Not like there's going to be the bird of paradise coming out of this remedy. Maybe small, pretty, little dainty flowers. It doesn't have a life span. You cut these flowers, the mistress will put them in the vase. After two days she'll throw them away.

The downside of this remedy: wilting; like a French mistress will wilt. It's decorative but it doesn't have strong roots. It has made me a tiny bit more domestic. I noticed I did the dishes twice and I usually don't do dishes.

Why the French mistress? Because they will do bare minimum, not going to be rolling up their sleeves and do the heavy-duty work. Like I said it's light, more carefree. I'm not as anal as I usually am.

This must be good for trauma people, for abused people. It doesn't retain. It doesn't allow you to fixate on any one thing. Not very passionate. Grey; doesn't mean murky but doesn't have very strong emotions either way. Good to give a bride before she gets married. Would eliminate the jitters. But it will retain its femininity.

Warps time; doesn't make you think of deadlines; **like time doesn't exist in a way.** Even if I'm late, usually if 10 minutes late I'm devastated. Not cutting, not critical. All will be well.

This isn't going to last long. I think I'll get bored. **Just skimming the surface**, not going to be satisfying. Gemini female; superficial, frivolous, very entertaining, they're making impressions & not trying to be negative, impressions of being carefree & lightheartedness. Images, not that they are like that, but this is how they project it.

Perfume – I always wear rose, softens my heart. Now I put on orange blossom. It's sweet; this remedy is sweetness.

This remedy you gave me is very much a café society; **skims the surface.** Pleasurable and light. Interesting to a certain degree. Sunlight'.

Comment (JS)
The image of a mistress is an interesting variation on the image of a teenager. She is carefree, colourful and lacks the heavy burden of the gray, adult responsibility that falls on a wife. Everything is taken care of, and all she has to do is play and enjoy the freedom, sunlight and sweet perfume of life!

CASE 13.9 3-year-old boy
Camilla Sherr, Tanzania

Male, age 3

First consultation
Mother: 'He is coughing half the night. I need long term treatment with him.

There's a new baby coming in January.

He is very dry. Mouth, lips, skin etc. He tastes very salty when you kiss him.

He doesn't pee much. He drinks a lot. He needs to pee but he doesn't want to, he holds it in.

He doesn't say what he wants. He will never say I want chocolate or anything. You have to guess.

He loves strawberries.

He doesn't have the urge to take what he wants or what he needs. As a baby he did not scream when he was hungry; he just accepted what is. He doesn't come out with it. He doesn't say.

He is very clever, very verbal, fluent talking when he was 1.5 years old.

He observes things, he is very abstract.

Also in the kindergarten, not easy for him to go into a game. Hard to take part.

Now he has fears.

Very fast thinking, makes many connections.

He is really into food. He likes to eat the spices, licking them, very interested in cooking.

He was born by C-section.

His mother had no milk, it took time, but **he didn't demand it. He waited patiently.**

He doesn't like if food is mixed together.

He loves bread. He loves food -Especially bread and beans, not sweets.

He is very clean, needs a napkin next to him.

Very tidy – a little bit compulsive. **If something is not in place, he hates it; he tidies things after his parents!**

Things need **to be closed** straight away after they are opened.

He doesn't want to wear shoes, barefoot all the time.

He doesn't like labels, I have to remove them.

He loves animals; loves cats, loves their puppy.

Reverse psychology works on him, he does the opposite. 'You cannot go in the shower', and he will.

He ignores people; he won't say his name to people.

It takes time for him to connect but when he starts to talk, he doesn't shut up.

He invents words.

He likes music very, very much. He chooses his music himself, Puts on the cd/s by himself.

He loves puzzles, books, music

He wakes up really hungry and cranky.

He is funny and witty! Calling people by their wrong names to be funny.

He is very obstinate.

If you don't cut the cucumber the way he wants it, he will become upset.

But he will not say anything!!!! He is so verbal, why won't he say??

He loves plants and herbs.

He has mostly adult friends; **harder to mix with other kids** in kindergarten. He does his own thing.

He loves tools. But he is not into cars, or anything with wheels.

He stopped diapers at 1.5 years, but didn't want to make his poo outside of the diapers, **he was holding and holding**, not agreeing to poo in the potty but not wanting diapers. He was really upset.

He got a remedy a year ago, every once in a while he asks for it; **Natrum muriaticum 200c.**

When he got it, it really helped him, it really cleared something, his sleep, his mood.

He doesn't get sick, no high fevers.

He laughs a lot. We can laugh about words. Humour from the beginning, loves a joke.

He doesn't like to go to other people's houses unless there is some interesting food there.

He was born by C-section, mother dilated very fast, 6 hours – very dilated, **but he wouldn't come down, he didn't flex**, he didn't put his head into the right position.

He was so quiet after birth. He was with his eyes open. Quiet.

He doesn't need; he isn't needy. Not even as a newborn.

Teething very late; first tooth at 9 months, still doesn't have the last 4, only has 2.

He doesn't show if he has a scratch. He will look sad – **but won't tell.**

He is so deep . . . out of my reach.

Dr Seuss, the Lorax – his favourite book; he knows the book by heart. Many details in one book.

He didn't connect to any doll, teddy or object.

Doesn't like meat.

He eats so neat and clean.

The beginning of pregnancy was so energetic, **I was flying**, so much energy.

As the pregnancy went along it became more and more physical, every time I took my remedy, Sepia, I would cry and I would dream all of us dying, every night someone else died.

Felt **my inner child was saying** you are doing such a stupid thing, emotional risk (dad died when I was 9).

For 6 months after he was born I was always waiting to find him dead. It took many months to release this fear.

Rx: Argon 200C

Follow-up 3 months
2 weeks a huge aggravation.

He wouldn't pee at all, it was coming out of his ears! We were cursing you Camilla.

He was so stubborn!

And then suddenly **he opened up.**

He just opened. It was beautiful.

He just let go.

He started peeing in the kindergarten.

He started playing with other kids which he never used to do.

Much more easy socially.

Suddenly crawling on the floor playing with other kids.

Big shift. Huge.

We feel he came into himself.

He is in his power now.

Improvement continues very nicely over the next two years. He does well on Natrum muriaticum in acutes.

Comment (JS)

The remedy was chosen in two stages. In the first stage a noble gas was indicated because of symptoms that are common to most nobles: not interacting, not demanding, not connecting. The inability to flex during birth and the tendency to hold on to urine and stool are also indications. We could say that he is self-contained.

Now to choose a specific noble. Indications for Argon are the love of jokes and humour, of music and play. His mother's feeling of flying in pregnancy and his love of plants and herbs (Day Three). He responds well to Natrum muriaticum, the closest remedy to Argon (see 'Related Remedies' in Chapter 16). Finally the tendency to be obstructed and then to suddenly flow relates to the passage from second to third dimension.

CASE 13.10 Imagine

Denise Straiges, USA

Female, age 13

First consultation
Preliminary conversation with mother:

Mum's biggest concern is that Libby is very physically guarded and doesn't let anyone get close to her. She doesn't want to be seen. Won't change clothes in gym class or in front of friends. Can't tell mum, "I love you." Also, that she's put on weight and has some acne.

Always liked playing on her own, especially engaged with music and reading. Was constantly loved and touched as a baby. Became more reserved after brother was born. Mum wondered how she could ever love a second baby and felt as if she betrayed Libby by loving her son.

Birth: The placenta didn't separate and mom was whisked away to surgery and thus, mom and baby were separated immediately upon birth. Libby never crawled as a baby.

Libby:

I saw a school counselor because I wanted to connect my physical and mental and not be all "up here" (Gestures with her hand above her head). I'm all thinking. I don't connect my head and body. I think a lot. More than I should. I daydream a lot.

I am Dylan-esque ... more thinking than doing. I don't live my life as Libby ... more like Bob Dylan and John Lennon did. I dwell on the '60s and '70s era.

In fourth grade there was a play on World War II and I sang, 'Imagine'. I was drawn to the chords. The picture on the album ... those eyes ... drawn to it. It was all I could think about: Lennon, Dylan, Springsteen, Joan Baez, Woody Guthrie. In fifth grade I took up guitar.

I don't feel like I have a group. I'm American, grew up in London, I like old music, I've been to seven schools. I realize I haven't been happy in a long time.

We moved back to America and right away went on a big holiday. We never got ourselves grounded. Started school and made a friend; after that I didn't feel alienated at all.

Not a day goes by when I don't think about London. What is everyone doing there? I've even stopped listening to music because it sounds weird now. Painful. I had such a good connection with London but left all that behind. It hurts to remember people's voices. I don't dwell in the past as much but it's still painful.

I get lightheaded quite often. I feel like I'm going to have a seizure. Bright fluorescent lights in school overwhelm my senses.

I am detached. I hold off a bit. Not rude, just not close. I keep people at an arm's length and don't let them into my spectrum of thinking. I've never had a best friend. I have always moved on. Probably because we moved so much.

I'm oddly afraid of chickens and bugs.

I like to watch shows about UFOs . . .

I'm anxious of outcomes and the future.

I don't have a purpose. I'm such an outsider.

I've missed out on the English childhood. And also the American childhood.

I've never had the same history as other people so I don't connect easily.

I rely on myself so I don't connect with other people.

I daydream a lot.

I'm always at the wrong place at the right time.

I went to NY for a weekend to wait for Yoko Ono.

John Lennon was connected. I'd love to be the reincarnation of him. Which leads to something I've been dwelling on. . . . I'm so much like him. Even my handwriting looks like his.

I'm dizzy and lightheaded since we arrived in America. I just want to collapse. Like I'm going to black out. It happens five times a day and is worse in school with the fluorescent lights. When I get up suddenly it's like a cloud comes over my head and I have to sit back down. It blocks out my senses. A harmonic tone. High pitched notes, floating, nausea.

Three summers ago had an awful ear infection and had to be in hospital for 3 days. Can't hear completely since. I get weird ear "tunings" like deaf people get. My vision is terrible but I don't wear my glasses since coming to America.

Major vertigo from my ears over my head. It's like my tuning is off.

Stomach: sharp pains (points above umbilicus) drawing in.

Periods are excruciating. Can't even move. Can vomit from the pain.

Sleep takes up to an hour and a half to fall asleep.

My guitar playing is a part of me that I think I've lost now. I write sad songs in minor chords. But nothing is coming anymore.

RX: Argon 200C, 3 doses in 24 hours

Follow-up 8 weeks
Playing music again. Listening to music again. Playing a lot of music. I'm obsessed with Coldplay and The Arctic Monkeys . . . but nervous to lose the John Lennon stuff. I already knew all there was to know, so now I realized I can expand my repertoire.

On the whole able to open up more on a whole different array of subjects. I used to be secretive about things to my mum; now I'm able to talk to her. I'm even comfortable changing in front of friends. And the chicken thing has gone away. No more vertigo or floaty feeling.

Have had really deep sleep.

Beautiful progress continued with intermittent doses of Argon 200C over two years. Libby continued to improve and during follow-ups reported meaningful shifts in her relationships, ability to communicate and overall physical health including sleep and menses. Mom, however, continually pointed out Libby's weight and "acne". An objective observation of Libby is that she is not at all overweight nor was there detectible acne beyond the usual "spots" of adolescence. Despite this, Libby was prescribed Acutane (a powerful acne drug linked to depression and suicide). Within a month of taking Acutane, Libby developed a deep depression:

"All my bonds were broken. I was so enveloped in my emotional state . . . it was like snow inside of me. Before, my inspiration was flowing but now I can never think of anything to say. I can't make decisions, I can't remember."

Towards the end of her six-month Acutane treatment she developed anorexia and began to exercise obsessively. When she came to a follow-up I didn't even recognize her.

Argon 200C brought back her periods (she had amenorrhea for nearly a year due to the anorexia) and she was beginning to experience a reduction in the disconnection and depression. Libby was then prescribed oral contraceptives and given the HPV vaccine and strong topical acne medication at which time she decompensated completely. Repeated doses of Argon ceased to touch the case at this point and no clear pattern had emerged to indicate the next appropriate remedy. Folliculinum 200C helped to establish some order in the case and shortly thereafter Argon 1M was given to great result.

"So good! Like the veil finally lifted again. I felt I could connect again. Could actually connect to people again. Interacting with people is much more natural. My hunger is regulating again and I actually felt normal hunger. I didn't have any PMS for two periods. A miracle!"

Explanation of analysis:

The verb of the case led me to the Noble Gas series (floating, detached, vertigo, not grounded, alien, sensorial aberrations). From there I considered the "locations" of the tension: From birth, the placenta didn't detach – resulting in separation from mum. And throughout Libby's life she has struggled to connect to others, which gives her pain. As this did not match the patterns I knew from study of Helium, Neon and Krypton, I looked at Argon relative to its place on the periodic table – in the row with Natrum, Magnesium, Silica and Phosphorus – remedies known for issues around establishment of identity and relationships. And finally, confirmation came in the signature of the remedy with fluorescent lighting exacerbating her vertigo.

The long-term evolution of this case (at this writing totals nine years) was particularly interesting in terms of management of the obstacles created by powerful, suppressive drugs (Acutane, oral contraceptives and the HPV vaccine). Ultimately, when Argon completed its action, Natrum muriaticum was indicated and a new level of healing reached.

Comment (JS)

Nice case. The main clue to Argon is the patient's yearning for the teenage years of our generation – Lennon, Dylan, Springsteen, Joan Baez, Woody Guthrie. Although she was not yet born, these artists are part of our culture's Summer of Love, the happy days of being an eternal child in a beautiful garden of love. Everything was perfect, people were together as one and teenagers blossomed in a flower power world. She felt she missed out on her childhood, and this was her way of replacing it.

Once she had the remedy, she moved on to a less childish era of Coldplay and Arctic Monkeys. The music was good but the dream was over and it was time for the 'eternal child' generation to grow up.

At the time of doing the case Denise did not have access to the Argon proving or book, so it is nice to see how her analysis dovetails with this information.

There are echoes of Natrum muriaticum all through the case: the sad music and keeping people away, not connecting etc. As we discuss later on, Natrum muriaticum is a sad echo of Argon, and they relate well to each other.

14

THE THIRD PERIOD

As if I am totally alone. Eight aspects of oneness, what I thought was one was a complete one, rather than eight fraction ones.

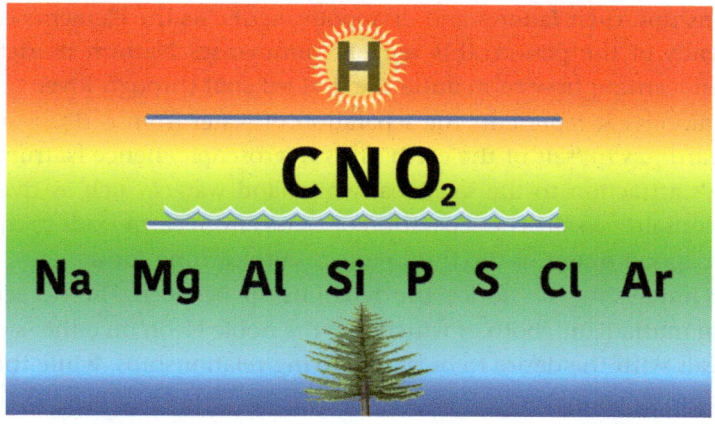

Figure 14.1 *First three periods of periodic table with the first three days or creation: Light, water, trees*

Argon is the culmination and perfection of the third period. By comparing the remedies of this row to Argon we can gain many insights into their individual characteristics and into the period as a whole. The following Argon symptom opens our exploration. It puzzled me for some time until its significance became clear.

Dream: a writer/sailor in bereavement whose life now divides in 3 – the 17% up front reclaimed, the 11% behind also coming out, the rest still in a shroud of swirling mists. I think 'Oh dear, not much real life in the percentages' and then I realise it is real progress.

This dream refers to the third period, elements 11–17. We are progressing towards Argon. The following periods are still hidden, shrouded in a mist.

The sailor travels the seas, which join the lands. He is in bereavement, and this brings us to our first remedy in the third period, Natrum muriaticum, the combination of elements 11 and 17. Just as the H2O molecule emulates Neon's ten protons and electrons, sodium lends its one spare electron to chlorine so as to mimic Argon's 18.

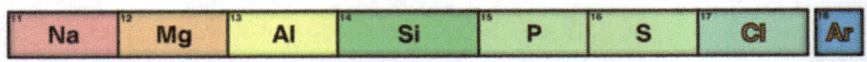

Figure 14.2 Third row of periodic table

Natrum muriaticum unites both extremes of the period, male and female, but their relationship is barren. It is a remedy that centres on loving relationships, their failures and disappointments. As the elements envelop both ends of the period, this remedy summarises Natrum muriaticum's essence: learning how to re-unite the divided soul through love.

Common salt represents the separation of water from earth. Salt represents earth, as in 'salt of the earth'. It is hygroscopic, hence Natrum muriaticum's attraction to the salty sea, while land waters, such as rivers and lakes, contain no salt. The separation of waters from earth leads to the great love disappointment of the third period, salt yearning for its sea.

It is interesting to notice the relationship between Fluoric acid and Natrum muriaticum, both of which hug the noble Neon on either side. The first deals with the desire to break up loving relationships, while the latter relates to the emotional consequences.

There are many well-known Natrum muriaticum themes that are reflected in Argon: the desire to be by the sea, the need to preserve the past, nostalgia, love disappointment, sad music, disillusionment, lump and dryness in the throat and constant sighing. Most prominent however is Argon's acute sense of grief.

The following symptoms of Argon are extremely similar to Natrum muriaticum, so spare a thought for Argon when you meet these situations in clinic. The differentiation may lie in the fact that Argon's grief stems from the loss of an ideal relationship, one which Natrum muriaticum can only yearn for, but Natrum muriaticum's love is often unrequited. While Argon seeks to preserve the perfect childhood and relationship, Natrum muriaticum preserves the imperfection of past disagreeable occurrences. When it comes to love and relationships, in the long-term Argon clings to the moment of perfection; the blossoming of teenage love, the perfect relationship, while Natrum muriaticum dwells on the near misses and 'could have been' relationships.

Expressions that are peculiar to Argon are **bolded**.

Right eye was closed, as if tears were lying **waiting for the sun to rise**.
Desire to go somewhere near the sea.
Love of the sea, better by the sea.
I felt very sad and tried not to cry but couldn't stop the tears flowing. I felt helpless.
Feel like weeping, but tears do not come.
Dreamt of feeling sadness when neighbour talked about my mother who had died.
Feeling depressed all day. Didn't want to communicate with anyone. Energy low – dragging myself around. Feeling unhappy and weepy.
Feeling tearful but cannot cry.
Felt extremely irritated but said nothing. Wanted to be left alone.
The words **'preservation'** and **'protection'** seemed to be significant.
Need to keep emotions hidden, as if only 1% exposed. Feels like the protection is not to show emotion.
Feeling of sadness and weariness.
Felt quite tearful and sad – **a sense of being suspended in some time zone where movements and actions are slowed down.**
Felt sad it is the **end of an era we are at now**. Nostalgic for the past, **an era is coming to the end with my parent's generation.**
Driving and scanning the music channel. Get a pipe lament and realise I have tuned into the Remembrance Day programme from England, I remember an uncle killed in the war and connect with my grandmother's anguish – it expands to the anguish of all mothers – a profound sadness engulfs me. Elgar's' music started and when the announcer began reciting a poem tears flowed down my cheeks. **I prayed fervently for world peace. I arrived at my destination at exactly 11.00 as the one-minute silence begins.**
Dream that my husband died. **We put him in a plastic bag and tied it at the bottom so that he was completely sealed in the bag.** We put him on a bed in a room. The next morning I found my small daughter fast asleep on top of him. The plastic bag was stuck to his face. [This was a terrible image. The grief I felt for days later was dreadful. Even though I was aware that it was only a dream and my husband was alive and well, I just could not be consoled. The grief was awful.]
I started thinking about the 21-year-old boy that was killed working on the sewage lying between my house and my old house. Last night it was. **A wall fell on him, like a lonely grave.** As I sat here, it seemed horribly sad. I haven't been able to get it out of my mind all week. Tears have just

welled up and I've been crying my eyes out. This was totally out of character for me. I don't even know who he was. It doesn't matter. This kid **being buried alive is like a monstrous disillusionment for a much younger self than my experienced old soul.** Weeping overwhelms me at the thought of the **beautiful illusion gone with this boy.**

I am not sure how I am in relationships. Am I safer for others if I am on my own. People were unavailable.

The sun plays a central part in Argon and Natrum muriaticum. The sun's ability to evaporate water or raise plant life lends Argon its vertical direction and third dimension. In Natrum muriaticum both the sun and its 11am zenith aggravate.

The sun's role is to unite the opposing forces of water and earth by evaporating sea into clouds that rain water on the earth, the water cycle. The heart of Natrum muriaticum is the sun, representing warmth and love. When the sun goes out of Natrum muriaticum's life through loss and grief, seas do not evaporate; rain and tears dry up and can no longer irrigate barren, deserted lands. The harmonious love of earth and water is disappointed.

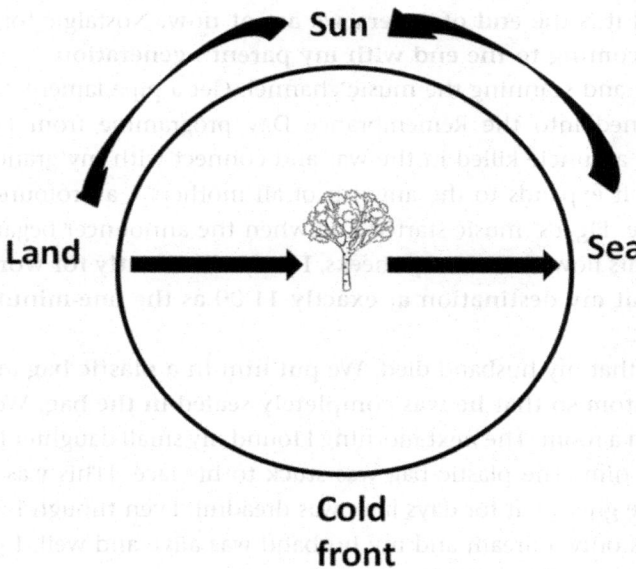

Figure 14.3 Sun uniting sea and land, the water cycle. No sun means no cycle

Angles of the third period

The upright man whose desires are good, wants the truth.
J.T. Kent

The theme of upright nobles occurs in Helium, Neon, Argon, Krypton and beyond. The following symptoms are proving expressions of seeing oneself from directly above or as being upright.

Feels as if I see myself from the outside and from above. (Helium)

Feel very tall, as though I am towering over everything. (Helium)

Sense that all limbs are foreshortened, my head and eyes feel huge, I feel as though I have eyes all over my head, that I am all-seeing. (Helium)

I feel invincible when upright. (Neon)

I now feel very upright in space and am aware that before, I was at a slight tilt – both physically and morally. The whole proving can be described as a rectification. (Neon)

A weight has been lifted, the bowed feeling has been replaced by uprightness. (Neon)

Felt like things were **uprighting**. I was **picking up** trees. (Argon)

Its ... about **angles and the shadows ...**, and the size of the shadow is in direct relation to **our angle**, our relationship to the sun. If the sun is **directly above**, there's no shadow. (Argon)

On waking I had a desire to cut the centre of my hair on the crown, so that it was sticking straight up, so that I could transmit as well as receive. (Krypton)

Sensation of feeling taller from crown of head upwards (Krypton)

Images of very tall elongated figures on going to sleep, similar to Giacometti sculptures. (Krypton)

Helium views the body directly from overhead so that they feel tall while the body appears foreshortened. When Neon is vertically aligned they are plugged in to infinite universal energy. Argon stands upright creating the third dimension and leaving no shadow, and Krypton is aligned with the vertical line of the present moment of Here and Now.

The concept of being upright and aligned is a 'family trait' of the noble gases, repeating in several of the group VIII remedies. In contrast, the 'ordinary' elements lean at various angles to the vertical axis of existence (Figure 14.4). They seek to rectify themselves to the perpendicular but can only do so by means of chemical interactions, in which they share electrons to mimic the noble uprightness. For example, picture the unification of the Natrum and Chlorum angles and you will get the perpendicular Argon.

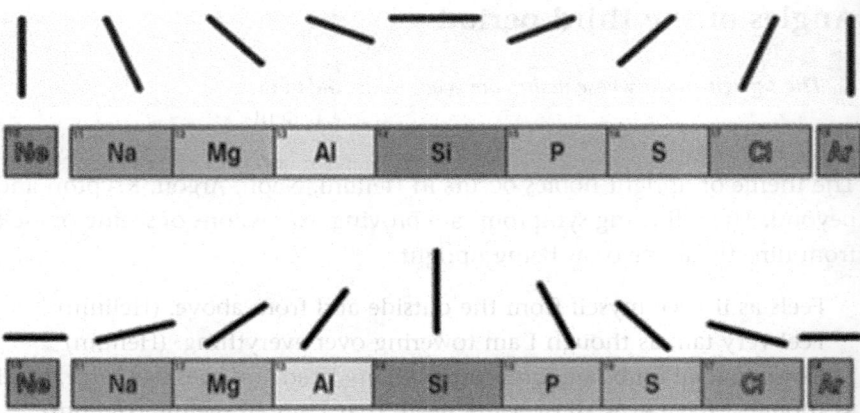

Figure 14.4 Angles of the third period. The bottom angles are perpendicular to the top ones

By studying the meaning of each noble gas's rectification, as achieved through vertical alignment, we can perceive its true nature and understand what the preceding period yearns for. Hydrogen lies in a horizontal line, spread across the universe and with no focus. It has lost its connection with the collective soul; therefore, it yearns to regain purpose through aligning itself with the individual, upright mission of Helium. Helium, however, is stuck in this vertical prison, unable to lean forward into life. Argon is represented by the upright tree forming a third dimension in space, and likewise it is analogous to the perfect young adult or the perfect relationship. The remedy Natrum muriaticum tries to mimic Argon but is unable to create the perfect relationship.

Each element forms a different angle to the upright noble. I arrived at the angles from dividing the straight line, which is 180°, into 8 (9 elements in the row including both nobles, with 8 spaces between them), which gives 22.5° between each element, as can be seen on the upper diagram in Figure 14.4.

Naturally this diagram is an analogy rather than a physical reality (as far as I know). The top diagram depicts the nobles as vertical, in their ultimate healthy and connected state, aligned with the universal force.

However each element or remedy holds within it the opposite and perpendicular state. The bottom diagram in Figure 14.4 shows the opposite, perpendicular state inherent in each remedy. At their worst, the noble gases become inert and prostrate, lying horizontally and thus cut off from universal energy and the purpose of life.

Here, Neon and Argon are shown in their flat state, as opposed to the aligned and electrified position in the top diagram. The centrally placed Silica is now vertical, like the sheath of wheat that can grow upright in health. It appears that, as in a sine wave, when Silica is healthy, the nobles are sick and vice versa. The reality is that each remedy carries both polarities at all times. Naturally the provings show both aspects of each remedy.[i]

As you will see from the mini provings below, these angles can shed some light on understanding the inner structure of the third period.

Meditation provings of remedies of the third period

The following are 'Mini Meditation' provings. Alongside the numerous full Hahnemannian provings Camilla and I have conducted, we have also experimented with meditation provings. The prover holds the remedy in their hand or sleeps with it under their pillow or uses similar means of proximity and induction. There are certain advantages to a mini meditation proving, provided that it is conducted with a highly sensitive person. It is quick and often brings out an unusual perspective. *It is essential that the prover be blind to the remedy.*

It is important to understand that such a proving can only offer suggestions for materia medica as an adjunct to full provings. The test is whether the symptoms match the totality and essence of the conventional proving, and whether they are borne out in clinic. Many of the meditation provings I have conducted alongside classical ones have proved their validity in clinic.

My wife Camilla, having participated in 17 Hahnemannian provings and having edited several more, has developed the sensitivity and acuity of senses to produce excellent mini meditation provings. She is quite clairvoyant, being born to a line of psychically sensitive people. Her meditation provings are unexpected, vivid and highly accurate. I particularly appreciate that, in contrast to many of the 'nicer' provings, she often reveals the 'negative' side of a remedy.

While these provings often seem to be in contradiction with the common essences, they are in full accord with the original provings. I am happy to do whatever I can to balance essences that are one-sided and distorted.

Note that some of the remedies, e.g. *Chlorum* do not appear in pure form in nature and hence these provings are unique in representing the pure element.

These provings were recorded verbatim from the moment they began.

---

[i] For further examples see Angles of the Materia medica. In: Sherr, J *The Dynamic Materia Medica of the Noble Gases: Neon.* Glasgow: Saltire Books, 2017.

Sodium Element 11

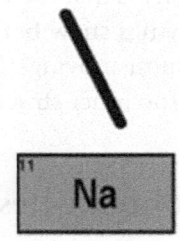

Figure 14.5 *Sodium*

Natrum muriaticum

The Joyful youth
Of Argon,
Cannot be recycled.
Lot's wife turns,
Craning neck
Attempting to preserve last
Memories of sin city,
Carefree days.
Preserved indeed;
Salt pillar freezing time,
Crystallising joyful moments
Into bitter recollections which
Cannot be grasped,
Sandy silicon grains slipping
Fingers,
The hour glass turns.

I feel like it is pushing me backwards, way back. (Leaning back.) *I want to do a backwards bridge.*

(Doing a bridge (yoga position). Bending backwards.)

The throat and neck, everything just wants to go back.

Like my head is loose and tipping backwards.

Back, back, back.

Neck pain (rubbing neck). *It's very, very strong.*

(Dipping head back while making a clicking sound. Constantly clicking and dipping head backwards.)

The axis is backwards, click backwards. I keep seeing the image of a hinge clicking backwards.

Now my back is arching backwards.

I just feel so tired of life, so tired.

(Crying)

Life is too exhausting. Why live, why bother, why try and try and try, what's the point? No point in anything, I don't know what the point is, so hard.

Life is so difficult. So much effort all the time. Just effort, effort, effort. (Crying while bending head back.)

Not happy at all. No joy in anything. (Grimacing and crying). *I used to be able to be happy about stuff and just enjoy little things. Now I don't have any, just depressed.*

Trying to make everyone happy and appease and manage everyone. All the time managing everybody and their emotions and shit and problems and heartache.

I just function for everyone else, doesn't matter what I want. What's the point, no point. I don't have energy for it.

No body understands me or gives a shit about me. I feel really alone and disregarded, part of the furniture. Who cares what I want. Even I don't. Completely lost my sense of who I am. I just exist for others, there's no me left anywhere.

If someone said, 'Go and do whatever you want,' I wouldn't have a clue what to do. Wouldn't be happy alone, wouldn't be happy with people. Not even that I feel like a failure, just feel like nothing. There is no me. Me, whatever that is, is not there.

Everything is hard, I'm exhausted.

I want to do stuff that matters. I feel I have no ego, no identity. So even if I could do anything I want, I wouldn't know what it was.

Pain in the groin left side, worse walking (New symptom).

Same feeling of head pushing back. Like neck clicking backwards.

(Sigh).

I feel worn out, shattered. I'm finished.

Oh God, I'm going to cry again.

All the joy being sucked out totally. Joyless, no joy left.

Image of an old drunk sitting in a restaurant by the pier watching the ships go by. He's feeling sad, doesn't give a shit. Nothing matters.

I feel Irish, like an Irish accent is coming on. A man sitting in a pub by the pier. I feel the corners of my mouth pulling down. Indifferent and sad and no enthusiasm or joy, no 'joie di vivre', sadness. Like you don't care any more. Sad because he can't go to sea any more, lost his mojo, and he knows there is nothing more for him, nothing left. You lose your point, you lose your Par 9, you don't even know what you want to do. If you do know, then you can't and you blame yourself, but if you don't know or lost mojo or too old or cripple or drunk, so get on that ship. It's so sad, such a sad place. Breaks your heart because you've lost it, can't get it back, too old, alcoholic or cripple. Either you had it and lost it i.e. can't do it anymore, or you lost it and don't know what it is anymore.

A very lonely place, so people come to you and say why don't you volunteer, or take a course in ceramics or go to the YMCA, but they don't get that there is no point in knitting for the sake of it. It won't do anything for a person like this. Like if I said to you, 'You know you must start sewing, because you've got nothing now. If you start sewing, it will help. But it won't, and you don't have a clue what you want to do. Writing a novel, living in Bali, learn Japanese, writing poetry, doing fuck all – you don't know what to do. So difficult to be in a good strong position when you don't have a fucking clue what you might want to do.

For these people, it's the most awful to get helpful suggestions from other people because nothing is going to do it. You have no sense of who you are, so how can you have a Par 9. You have to know a little bit of who you are to have Par 9 Because how will you know what moves you. You have no sense of who you are You don't know if you want to be with people or work with computers or teach or be an engineer or researcher or economist. To make any of those decisions you need some kind of a sense of who you are, so everything is pointless.

Either you had it and lost it or never had it. Much worse if you had it and you lost it and people say you can't be a sailor anymore, so now let's work out Plan B. But the captain is who you were and it made you happy, and now you have to do something different that doesn't pan out. The saddest thing is to retire from something you love and to have nothing left.

Comment (JS)

We see the angle of Sodium being pushed backwards, just as in Camilla's proving. A moment ago, it was in the perfect vertical alignment of Neon, and therefore connected to its purpose in life, Paragraph 9. But that has now passed, and like the ageing Neon (Neon is water) sea captain, he can no longer fulfill his mission. He can only sit in a pub by the shore, look back with regret and mourn his loss.

Magnesium Element 12

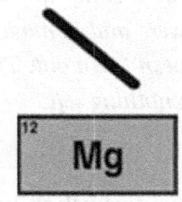

Figure 14.6 *Magnesium*

Magnesium and friends

Water bed, months nine
Now I'm ready, quite sublime
Nourished at my mother's breast
Chocolate sister do your best
Feed until I have my fill
Just like brother chlorophyll.

I burn so bright, I love to fight
And so I lose my friends
But when the quarrel's over
I have to make amends.

With cousin Phos I'll cramp your style
With aunty Carb I'm sour
But I'm forsaken on my own
I need my parents and a home.

So love and nourish, mom and pop
Carry me and please don't stop
For if you quarrel or don't smile
You'll get a baby Chamomile.

(After one minute.)

(Eyes crossing over.) *I feel cross-eyed but more rolling over backwards.*

Wow! Oh God, God!

(Sighing forcibly.)

I feel like I'm doing summersaults backwards. My eyes are rolling backwards, my whole being is rolling backwards.

Oh God, I feel like I'm curling over backwards, rolling in backwards circles.

I can hardly keep my eyes open.

I feel like a leaf, like a fern, but not curling forward, rather curling backwards.

(Laughing)

It's like yawning is part of curling backwards.

I feel my whole face is pulling downwards, like the corners of my mouth are going down.

I really feel like gravity is pulling me down, pulling my cheeks down, like gravity got hold of me.

Will I never be able to smile again? What a pull down.

(Mouth corners pulled down.)

Trying to pull lips up.

If this is permanent I will kill you! (Laughing)

Oh my God!

I am so tired, I feel like gravity is pulling down my eyelids. Like gravity got hold of me, just pulling me down. Every part of me is so heavy. Oh my God, my eyes are so heavy!

Falling asleep. I feel super heavy. My eyes are so heavy.

(Observation: She is talking as if from a dream.)

I feel like I'm younger. I am little but they want big things from me and I am not managing to do them. I am making excuses saying I couldn't because of such and such. A feeling I can't do it, I'm too young. What is asked from me is too much; I don't know how to do it. All the time it's a feeling of failure. Falling asleep and feeling I am not doing this properly, messing it up, but feel too heavy, like drugged.

Whenever I close my eyes, they feel like rolling back in their sockets.

Something about people staring and looking and not being good enough.

Dreaming someone trying to convince someone else with more authority. Always uneven situation, where we are lower or not good enough and have to explain ourselves, but it doesn't go anywhere.

Feels Like WWI or WW II maybe, in the dream. Someone's mother in the first war, trying to get out, but this person is blocking the energy.

Then there was someone else trying to block us. I don't know who she is. Like we were trying to flee, get on a plane and trying to flee Nazi Germany. Someone driving a car and they get stopped by the police and they want to see inside the bags. And they show all these electrical little wires, trying to convince them there is nothing dangerous in the bag and trying to get away.

Many little snippets of dreams but I can't grab them properly. I can't understand what I'm doing wrong. Like all the time failing, failing, failing. Nothing is working out. Bizarre – nothing working out in the dreams. (I ask: 'Dreams unsuccessful'?) *Yes.*

(Mouth corners pulled down sharply.)

All the time different little dreams, exhausting me.

I feel I'm not doing a good job.

I feel like a refugee.

In the dream I see many, many different people. I am trying to go somewhere or reach somewhere or explain something and it doesn't work out. In all these situations I was young and at the mercy of others and people had to do it for me. I could not do it myself.

How young? 11, maybe 12, 10–12, before puberty, before 13. You don't have the tools, not equipped, don't know how to do it.

I am somehow powerless. I can't do it on my own. I don't know how to do it, cause I'm just 11 or 12. I can't do it, I don't know how (a wimpy childish voice).

(Didn't anyone show you how?)

They are not doing it well. I am not getting to where I need to go. I need to run away. Something bad is going to happen and I have to get away. But they are not doing it well and I can't get on that boat, and I don't know how to do it alone, a frustrated helpless feeling where you are failing.

Like a government or Nazi or something big and you have to leave. You know you have to leave but you don't have the tools to know how. An impotent feeling, both in emotions and dreams. I am actually crying now. I feel really bad. If someone would just come and say, 'Come with me, we are getting on that boat', it would be OK. But no one is coming, only incompetent adults and they can't get it together, no one in charge to show the way.

I feel like am an orphan. I'm alone, no parents, all these people trying to help are strangers. I feel like I'm at their mercy. Not one there for you, no one doing the adult stuff that needs to be done. I can't do it, I don't know how to do it. Frustrating.

The rolling backwards, maybe I went back in time. I was pushed backwards . . . rolled me backwards.

Also, I feel like I'm on the Titanic. Had a vision of being on the Titanic, same feeling. It's sinking and nothing you can do, impotence. No one can save you and you can't save yourself. I feel very, very sad. It feels like the end is coming, and I don't know how to stop it. Want to give up, it won't happen, I won't be saved. I do not know how to save myself, don't know what to do.

(Observation: She is crying, sobbing, whimpering like a child for several minutes. It took me some time to calm her down and tell her Mummy and Daddy were there, till she felt she got on the boat.)

(After being told what the remedy was . . .)

This is like a child of a Chocolate, who thinks he is ready to leave and can be on his own, but doesn't take responsibility, not ready and still needs parents very much.

The parenting of this day and age is shit. People give their kids too much choice and they can do anything, and no one really cares and makes an effort for you. Children must feel people care around them. Too much looseness and freedom is not good at all. Those poor kids in Auschwitz and all the concentration camps where they lost their parents, so terrible.

Too small, still incompetent and helpless. Can't deal with a big thing, Nazi or Titanic, very existential.

Comment (JS)

Looking at Magnesium's angle in the upper diagram of Figure 14.4, we see a line tilted backwards at 45^0, even further backwards then Natrium. It is midway up, but unable to stand up completely, hence it falls back as in the proving. Magnesium is half-way to standing on its own two feet, but cannot quite make it beyond childhood to a vertically upright adult. He can deal with small issues but is unable to rise to face grown-up size problems, and so he falls back. This is the orphan, no parents or guardians to teach him how to deal with the big stuff like war or the Titanic. Element number 12 is like a 12-year-old on the threshold of adulthood, but with no one to guide him through the difficulties.

Magnesium plays a very important role in the development of plant roots, and is absorbed through them. When a child is brought up with good guidance and parenting, they can develop strong roots that enable them to face the bigger problems in life. The magnesium remedies lack these roots due to poor or no parenting; hence they are unable to withstand the pull of gravity. The result is helplessness and unsuccessful efforts, as can be seen in the proving and the magnesium dreams.

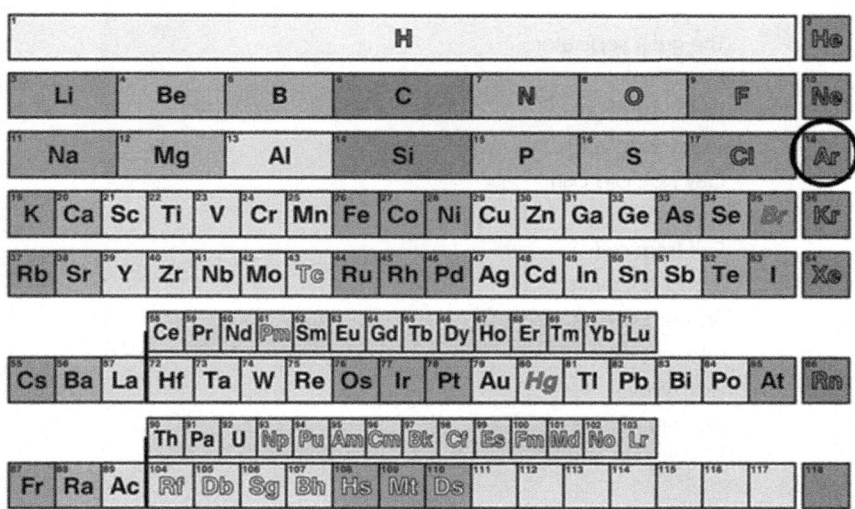

Figure 14.7 Periodic Table showing position of Third Period elements

Aluminum metallicum Element 13 and Alumina Al_2O_3

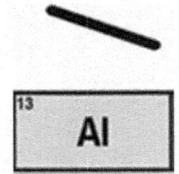

Figure 14.8 *Aluminium*

Alumina

The great separator
Cleaving
Earth from water
Water from earth
Clay pot, old pan
Knife carving
Self from self
Blood dripping
Severed nerves
Old and new
Fast, slow
Who am I?

(After one minute.)

When I look at you (JS), I am having thoughts of you as a baby, a cute little moochy-koochy baby, and then metamorphosing into an adult. Seeing you beyond all your bullshit, straight into you, like looking into your eyes and seeing the real you behind it all. Behind the layers and layers of thought and beliefs and disappointments and ideas and baggage, all the debris we accumulate over a lifetime, a glimpse of pure you. That's why babies are so attractive, no baggage, you see the real of who is there, who's at home.

What I saw in you from the first was something pure and clean, not the usual debris and shit and flotsam, all the accumulated crap, which is the opposite of the purity of the soul. That is why sex is so important, because it's a connection to the purity, and it should be regularly on the agenda, even if one doesn't feel like it. Once you start, it is fun, and it should not be left unattended for too long. It's a health and spiritual issue, fundamental.

We need to come from a zero place where we want nothing, the baby in us, not the place of wanting more. Like people are when you give them the little finger and they want the whole hand, always want, want, want: food, drink, information, chocolate, more, more, more, why always more? It's not the place of purity.

This is about connecting to the pure in you, the pearl in you. You take care of it and cherish it and look after it. The pearl is the purity in you.

The reason sex is so important is because in that moment all the shit vanishes momentarily and you connect with the real person, beyond the person's acquired layers. If there is no sex you only deal with the debris on the surface, the flotsam and the beliefs and shit we identify with, which has nothing to do with the real truth, just the little truths we chose to believe in. That is why so many marriages fail. If you only look at the debris, why would you want to stay married, just discussing work and little things that are completely beside the point. That is why people have affairs, just so they can have a real connection with someone's real self, past the shit that floats around the persona. We believe in the shit and flotsam and the rubbish, we buy into it. That is why we need sex and meditation, to connect with YOURSELF and forget about your debris for a while.

(She starts to cry.)

The fact is that there is so much perfection and beauty and love and beautiful souls around us. We have it all, we really have it all, but instead of focusing on the perfection and purity and beauty at the core of what we have, we just look at the debris and shit and accumulated baggage, how we think we want it. We just see the faults and the lacks and what is not. We don't connect with what is pure. (All said while crying in a childish voice.)

It's a real shame, you walk through life and don't see and don't appreciate what you have, just want more, more, more, a different thing or project that will somehow fulfill you. But it never, ever will crack it. The only way to be happy and fulfilled is to connect to the source and soul and all the perfect souls around us. But we just criticize all the time. It's a crime to do that. It's like spitting God in the face. Look at your children just a moment before they wake in the morning, and see the perfection and beauty and how much you love them and the perfection you and they are. Remember how precious they are, just a moment where you cherish them before you wake them and the shit begins.

It's the part that connects with God, that is God in us that every person has. It's all around us, in us. It's there all the time, but the light gets hidden behind all the garbage. You have to see it, all the beautiful moments and seconds and glimpses everywhere. It's so abundant, in our face all the time, but we don't see it. If you only focus on what is lacking, it's harder to see it.

To say to every person, 'I see the perfection that you are'. Connecting with the potential of absolute perfection that is in everyone. If you walk around life really believing that everything is perfect and right, even the shit becomes perfect, because you connect to it and see God through everything. You can even be married to an asshole and think that it is good, because you see the beauty in them, the God in them, and disregard the crap and issues, the dirt and beliefs we create every day; stuff like, 'I must write my books, I must be skinny, I must cook three meals a day, I must not waste time, do this and that and the other', and we buy into all this. It doesn't matter one bit what we do, but how, how we live our life. The only way to paddle through the shit is to connect to the perfect imperfection that is you, to the God in everything. Every day we should pray and thank God, and then you put the God in yourself first and can be satisfied. Otherwise you just climb into the tree like a baboon with your ass first. Meditation, sex and God are the answer.

I don't know why it makes me cry so much. Seeing the world from this perspective is not a gift or talent, it's something you can practice. Instead of teaching maths at school, there should be lessons in this, something you can learn so it becomes automatic. This remedy is a bit childlike, so basic and simple, and maybe kids do it, something naïve about it, so simple, no clever philosophy about it, you can't make money from it, just create people that are content.

Physically I felt very fat in the middle, like big boobs hanging on lards of fat underneath. Plump and benevolent.

Comment (JS)

From Kent's *Lectures on Materia Medica*, Alumina:[1]

This remedy comes in very nicely after Alumn (Alumen-JS), which has much Alum. in its nature and depends largely upon Alum., which is its base, for its way of working. It occurs to me to throw out a little hint. When you have a good substantial proving of an oxide or a carbonate, and the mental symptoms are well brought out, you can use these, in a measure in a presumptive way, in prescribing another salt, with the same base, which has a few mental symptoms in its proving. For instance, you have a group of symptoms decidedly relating to Alumn. The mental symptoms of Alumn., however, have not been brought out to any extent, but still you have the mental symptoms of the base of Alumn., which is the oxide, so that if the patient has the mental symptoms of Alum. and the physical symptoms of Alumn., you can rationally presume that Alumn. will cure because of the Aluminum in each.

As always, Kent in his genius depicts the essential feature of a remedy with a little story. Every time I read this paragraph, I end up confused about who is who and what is what; Alum, Alumina, Alumen, the oxide, the metal etc. This paragraph is a good example of the confusion of identity typical of the alums. As Kent says, it is difficult to separate their individual characteristics, and it is easy to cross their identities.

The well-known confusion of identity of Alumina is well represented in Camilla's proving. At the core of our being is the pure and essential Identity we are born with. But with time this purity is covered with an accumulated myriad of personas, beliefs, desires and aversions that we falsely believe are our real identity. These are however only the murky personas we have created from the sum of our acquired life history, an accumulation of stronger dissimilar experiences.

In Taoist practice the pearl represent our core inner identity, which we strive to clean and polish so that it shines through all the debris.

Extracts from Vermeulen's *Synoptic Reference 1*, Alumina.

(Bold highlights are by JS)

Alumina is pure clay . . . Nature seems to expect aluminium to remain clay. **The metallic condition is unnatural for it, the metal is not only difficult to extract, but the extraction would immediately be undone** if a peculiar circumstance did not protect it from attack. Like impenetrable armour, aluminium oxide immediately covers the metal with a fine protective layer of patina, 'noble rust'.

Aluminium is capable of taking brilliant polish and retaining it in dry air. In moisture, an oxide film forms. This protective layer seals off oxygen, thus preventing further oxidation. Although it is only 0,0001 millimetre thick, few chemicals can dissolve this colourless, tough and non-flaking film. Without this protective film aluminium would flare up even in the air and burn with a blinding flame.

It has been suggested that Alumina is the 'stuff' from which man was created[i]. From the proving of Oxygen,[ii] we have learnt that this remedy represents ego, greed and neediness. Just like pure clay, we cannot retain the purity of our simple and beautiful core but are immediately covered by the protective layers of oxygen ego. As soon as we outgrow the naivete of babyhood, or as soon as we wake in the morning, we cover ourselves with this oxidative rust. Without this layer we would burn pure and bright; with it we lose our pure identity. We live as a contaminated aluminium oxide rather than the pure aluminium metallicum.

Psora begins with the first breath of oxygen, when the midwife declares, 'It's a boy!' or 'It's a girl!' We gain identity and lose purity. Alumina is a primary psoric remedy, and is bold type in the most primary psoric of all rubrics, 'Itch without eruption'. It belongs to the early stages of life.

Note the angle of Aluminum in the upper diagram in Figure 14.4. It depicts an early stage of just beginning to rise from the horizontal. This is reflected in the early life, baby stages of acquiring identity and the symptoms on waking and rising in the morning.

On the other extreme, when this ego becomes fixed and hard it evolves into sapphire, a gemstone composed of aluminum and oxygen (Al_2O_3) and one of the most judgmental and avaricious remedies in the materia medica. And while this gem has its beauty, it has lost the simplicity of its inner clay. Oxygen prevails. As a gem stone, we see its opposite angle, standing at 90 degrees to the first, a near noble vertical line.

Aluminium has been detected in the brain cells of patients with Alzheimer's disease, but it is not known whether the metal's presence is a cause or an effect of the disease. Likewise, Down syndrome babies have higher levels of aluminium in their brains.[3] Probably associated with high aluminium concentrations in the brain as well, is, the neurological syndrome dialysis dementia that occurs in some long-term dialysis patients.[4]

The toxic aluminium, which is found in pots, building materials and vaccinations confuses our being and brain, leading us to an existential state of Alzheimer's in which we totally forget who we really are. But long before such a pathology flowers into its tragic end result, we are already lost in

---

[i] In multiple origin stories, man is made from clay. Scientists theorize that the minerals in clay lead to formation of proteins, DNA and living cells. (See *Mail Online.* 5th November 2013. Available online at: https://tinyurl.com/yccftw2)._

[ii] See Oxygen. In: Sherr J. *The Dynamic Materia Medica of the Noble Gases: Neon.* Glasgow: Saltire Books, 2017.

the multitude of identities we have created rather than remaining in the purity we were at birth, the moment before we awake and cover our true selves with the debris of life.

To sum up, Aluminum and its oxide are steps in the third period's progression towards Argon, from child to adult. Pure Aluminum lives in the purity of childhood, whereas Alumina is the development of ego and false identity that represent one step down the line towards adulthood.

Relevant rubrics (*The Complete Repertory*)[5]

Agriculture, inaptitude for

Ailments from sexual desire, suppression of

Anguish, morning, awakening

Confusion of identity

Confusion of mind, morning, waking on, rising amel

Delusion, as if someone else said it when he did

Delusion, money, delusion counting money

Delusion, possessed

Delusion, something behind him,

Dementia, in old people

Discontent with everything

Itch, without eruptions

Mathematics, algebra, geometry, inept for

Recognize does not, oneself, in the mirror

Placement on Circle: Earth – Water axis.

We mold clay by adding water.

Silicon Element 14

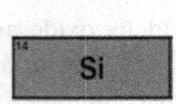

Figure 14.9 Silica

Silica

Seed bursts, now ready
Germinating, sprouting
Pushing sunwards
Poised to penetrate
Earth barrier

Sheath forming
Tip pointing
Gathering strength
Gaining length
I pierce
Then retreat.

First reaction, my mouth went into a smile but a very wide straight smile and a hum, like emmmm, all good. Yes, yes all good hmmmm emmmm. Making positive sounds with a permanent smile. All good hmmmmm. Laughing.

A straight horizontal smile without showing teeth. (Laughs) *Oh my God.*

Oh God, I feel like an American that walk around with a permanently satisfied smile, but it feels real. . . . I feel happy, mellow, nothing is problem. Saying 'I'm Positive' in an American accent, but I'm not faking it, feel like a positive person. I have a positive outlook. Everything is good, God is good, the universe is good. Awesome!! (mimicking American accent)

If you had that smile all the time, you would never get wrinkles.

Someone which makes positive lip sounds mmmmm emmmm emmmmm, smile, not an open smile – closed lips, like an annoying therapist. Eh hmm ehhmm, mmmm. You know there can be a whole mmmmm language like this without speaking.

(She starts talking in mmmm emhmmm language, making a whole sentence, mmm in different intonations. This goes on for a while.)

Like content people who sit in front of the fire with a cup of tea, all peaceful and quiet. Like XX, this is her remedy. She is lovely but I hate her. She looks you in the eye and goes mmm emmmmm, and is always positive. Very irritating. She teaches nonviolent communication. Mmmm mmmm. Very nonviolent, like a whale or dolphin, very nonviolent, no fuck words. Oh God, save me from such people.

Oh, I would be such a nice person if I was like this, big eyes, compassionate look, mmm mmmm, tilt your head a bit. No teeth to bite with. No teeth to bite – maybe they don't exist – the teeth.

Very passive, non-confrontational feeling, content, satisfied, quiet, definitely not argumentative. So much compassion and empathy, it's oozing out. It makes me really appreciate who I am. I would shoot myself if I was like that. Maybe in another 800 lifetimes I can be like this. I never want to evolve, prefer to be like I am, not all mmmm mmmmm.

But it doesn't feel fake. It's very easy to do non-violent communication; you can make 800 dollars an hour by teaching others how to hum. This is a pacifist's remedy in the purest way, not aggressively marching against wars. This is truly non-aggressive, truly love and peace, like a real hippy, the real McCoy. They don't believe in it, they are it. Mmmmmmm – smiling with mouth closed. If I do it to you all day, let's see how violent you become. Ha Ha.

I can't stop the smile. It's very straight horizontal mouth closed. Really someone who receives. They are not actively pushing anyone's buttons. They just mmmm away in understanding. You can't react because there is nothing to react against, just pure acceptance and compassion and receiving. A low vibration mmmmm.

Not a verbal remedy, can't express herself in words. The vibration is like a whale that communicates with hums or songs, vibrational communications. Like a different language. Before language was developed maybe people communicated like this, mmmmm emmm. It comes from the abdomen. These people are frustrating to deal with as they can't express their feelings. The language center not too well developed. Can't put thoughts into words. Feels like they communicate old information, like an old rock deep in the earth. Every time I want to communicate, I start humming. A vibrational communication.

Other people are animated when they speak, waving their hands, changing their words and voice – a huge scale of communication. This is very different, they are just OMmmmm, versions of OM coming out, very few notes. Connects to an ancient good part in us, good, service, serving people. No ego, the ego is not developed, like before ego. Harmony and nonviolent communication. OM – a vibration. When you do Om mediation it puts you in a place where these people already are. The OM cleans you out of words, to just be. Very powerful, when you are with people like this your whole frequency becomes lower, very calm.

A smile but lips don't go up, don't laugh like crazy, not higher frequency or high pitches or giggle. Just emmmm, not show teeth. Maybe it's about not baring your teeth. You can't bite, not confrontational. Good way to put yourself to sleep. Lower your vibrations and by going humming mmmmmm. Like ultimate yin, all yin, no yang. Yang didn't come, yang stayed behind. Ultimate female energy, totally round.

The weakness is that it is very difficult for them. To get up and go would be very hard, very difficult to make decisions. Like when in dangerous situations they would not flee or run, just be slaughtered without any resistance. Teaching would be difficult for them. Articulating – putting thoughts into words, I keep thinking of a whale – wise and old, but not savvy, not street-wise. For people in monasteries or spiritual communities of likeminded people or hermits. Can't communicate verbally. Mercury has a huge influence in this age – communication and internet and messages, quicksilver, very fast. These are very slow, would not be able to deal with mercury energy. They ponder each word before they say it. It has to be very accurate. Once you say it is out of your mouth; opposite of mercury in every way. Slow remedy, can be a big disadvantage. Can't get up and go. People who connect to stones.

*Often therapists, they would not be a talker in consultations, just nod and smile
and say a word here or there. Or autistic Asperger people who can't communicate
in words.*

Comment (JS)

Once again, an extremely accurate proving. This is Element 14, pure Silicon,
and not the SiO_2 of our materia medica. This purity shines through the
proving.

As we can see from the upper diagram in Figure 14.4, Silica is in the
middle of the period and at its worse it lies horizontally, like Camilla's horizontal smile. This angle is reflected all through the proving. It will have
difficulty standing up. It will have difficulty getting going or pushing out
a thorn, no 'Get up and go', no yang power. Silica will not stand up for
himself. As Kent puts it:

> What Silica is to the stalk of grain in the field, it is to the human mind. Take the
> glossy, stiff, outer covering of a stalk of grain and examine it, and you will realize
> with what firmness it supports the head of grain until it ripens; there is a gradual
> deposit of Silica in it to give it stamina.[6]

The wheat will not grow upwards without Silica's curative powers. The horizontal, toothless smile is an accurate sign – no bite and slow, difficult
teething. In its opposite mode, as shown in the lower diagram of Figure
14.4, Silica will be vertical, like a healthy stalk of wheat. These two opposite
angles signify either pure strength or pure weakness. This is its signature:
Silica is a semiconductor – flow or not flow, yield or be obstinate, penetrate
or retreat.

The vibrational aspect is another key factor in Silica. Quartz or silicon
dioxide SiO_2 is one of the most common minerals on Earth. Quartz oscil-
lates at a precise frequency of 32,768 times each second. It is this property
that allows it to be used in clocks and computers. The proving describes
someone like a rock, lying deep under the ground, who cannot rise upwards
and can only communicate by oscillating, but who is at peace.

As in Camilla's description, Silicon Valley is full of genius Asperger types
who are very positive and clever but cannot express themselves properly.

Finally and remarkably, Silica is an inimical remedy to Mercury. It is very
clear from the proving how these two substances have totally opposite
energies.

Phosphorus Element 15

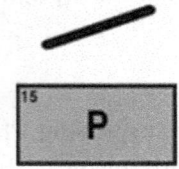

Figure 14.10 *Phosphorus*

Phosphorus

Don't focus on the sweet diffusion
That's a one-sided delusion
Clairvoyance and sympathy
A fraction of this remedy . . .

Nitro Mother
Sulphur brother
Silica sister
Magnesium lover

With such a charming family
You'd hope for love and harmony
But Phos can only feel disgust
And cheerful animosity

This remedy which seems so nice
Can also murder with a knife,
Hates mankind and company
Loves abuse and vice

Un-lucky element one-three
From fertilizing ATP
Causes very rapid growth
Emaciation and TB
Fatty liver, Kidney leak
Bloat anemia and dropsy
Mucous membrane, blood disorder
Seeping through an ulcered border

(After one minute.)

I feel my lungs. I can't get enough air; my lungs are constricted. Like I can't breathe deep enough; bra feels too tight.

Can't get enough oxygen into my lungs.

(Breathing faster and more shallow. Deep sigh.)

Can't pull the air in properly. It's stuck in my upper chest and not going all the way down.

(Undoing bra. Opening the window.)

Almost shaking like a panic attack, can't breathe. It's horrible.

Breathing deep, I going to faint! Standing by window. Having a panic attack, going to cry!

Fuck, I'm going to faint. Trying to breath. I am going to cry. This is horrible, fuck! Pulse is beating fast.

I can't get enough air.

(Drinking water in one large gulp.)

Deep breathing. I was shaking, really trembling, I could not breath. That was nasty!

(Lying down and covering head in blanket.)

(Moaning) *Ahh ohhh. I'm cold, I am really cold!*

I feel really sorry for myself. Why did you do this to me? I am going to cry!

Fuck you. I'm not doing this again. I don't like it.

Give me the diamond you owe me. I'm not doing anything ever again until you give me the diamond you owe me. (Breathing deeply.)

Like I can't get enough air.

I really want to be outside.

I feel very grumpy and sorry for myself.

I feel like a grumpy child want to scowl mouth (puckering lips).

I want to hug a teddy bear, to feel very sorry for myself. I want to be left alone.

I feel very cross with the world, like they have done something to me. The world owes me, I am owed something by the world and they are not giving it to me.

Body scattered on the bed
Decomposing into death
Necrosis oozing into bone
Ghosts invading haunted home

Fat and thin, red and white[i]
Tall and short, milk and spice
Divided forces dark and light
Tell a tale of fire–ice

Lightning flash, Thunder strike
Death dispersing into life
Light and dark, world war two
Hamburg burning[ii] German Jews[iii]

Deadly fight, day and night.
Porous border
Of Twilight

Feel like a petulant child that doesn't get what she wants.

Give me my stuff, you owe me.

People who feel they are owed something, not getting what they should deserve.

Even the air, why am I not getting the air owed me.

You don't get what you are owed – give me my money, my teddy, my diamond, you owe me, or I will do nothing. I'll just lie here.

Why should I do anything for anyone if the air I am breathing is not enough.

I don't get something so I am not giving anything back!

(Sigh)

The air is not enough.

No satisfaction that you are getting what you need. You feel you deserve more and should get it and no one giving it to you, like not enough air.

It's like the giving and receiving is completely out of balance.

I feel like someone who gives nothing and who wants everything. Or gives nothing without something in return.

I would never just give. Just give me something back. Why should I give otherwise? What's in it for me?

No one giving me enough so why should I give. Not even enough air to breath, so what does anyone want from me? I won't give nothing, they can fuck themselves!

I will never give any of our money to anyone again, our money is safe!

It's quite nice to be like this. Laughing, fuck them all! Never give anything for free any more.

I keep feeling my lungs, the main part of it – it's the oxygen and carbon dioxide interplay.

If you can't get enough oxygen, you can't give CO_2.

It feels like this is the beginning of all exchange and all bartering. All the 'I get this and give you that', the first giving and receiving.

But it's not receiving and giving harmoniously. It is about getting and not giving back, grabbing. I don't want to give back. I am not getting enough O_2 so don't want to give, but I have to, so resent it. It's all about balance of plus and minus.

I want to vomit – an urge to vomit. It's about getting something out. It's about grabbing and holding on, but something has to come out, so give vomit.

I feel like a really selfish bastard, low-life prick. It's all about the money, the balance. I get this much oxygen, that's what I give back, not one iota more. Like a pit that cannot be filled.

Not having enough or be satisfied. Nothing is enough.

It's all about me. Me, me, me, me, me, and others exist to fill me.

This person would not do voluntary work or give for the sake of giving or have a consciousness of give or receive. Always a feeling of lack, such a fundamental lack that I can't give, a miser, the ultimate avarice.

Not someone who hordes because they want more, just not enough. Not enough so you need to get more.

Maybe a shopaholic, shop moments. You feel gratification from buying but then comes feeling of lack. The spending is self-fulfilling.

Fundamental emptiness not filled. It seems lungs are too small and can't take in enough oxygen.

I feel like a victim, like I have been done in and not getting enough. Who did this to me, pissed off and angry and grumpy.

I don't feel empty, but the vessel is not big enough, like my lungs don't expand. Can't get enough air and air is money. Your first breath and need is air. Before food or drink or anything else, you need air, your most basic need. So if not enough air, you will never feel good. Food and drink is a luxury. It's like being robbed of your birthright.

You cannot trust the universe to provide you with enough. If there is not enough air, with every breath you are not getting enough. Every molecule someone not giving me is taken away from me. The energy is not flowing and exchanging and moving and transforming. It's stuck and cannot turn into benevolence and love and giving. The transformation from O_2 to CO_2 doesn't happen properly, so I feel everyone is stealing from me and I am not going to give them.

Give me my diamond!! You owe me!

I now understand the dragon in the mountain with the hobbit. The dragon is lying on a mountain of gold and it still wants more because is not enough. It's not filling the hole, except its need for oxygen. Maybe it's burning up all the oxygen with its fire.

My prices are going up and no more free treatment!

(Sighing deeply)

A horrible nasty feeling of lack.

It doesn't matter how much you make, it will never feel like you have enough. The dragon on the gold; you feel everyone is thieving. People are thieves!

This person never has enough; fundamentally deprived. Nothing will be good, and it's awful but all about oxygen. If you robbed from air, it's translated into money.

Also for people who spend a lot of money, because you have a feeling of lack. So sporadically this person will spend and spend and buy, buy, buy because temporarily it makes you feel satisfied and full, but then comes the hangover and you don't have enough.

It can be sporadic giving. In moments you get enough air and feel momentarily full, so you can give. Even these poor people can give something. It's not really good, like vomit, like bulimic people who eat and eat to feel full but then have to give back with vomit. Not stingy by nature, just lack.

This is physical. Started with a panic attack that can't breathe, no oxygen. Then came the absolute feeling of, 'You owe me. Give me what you owe me, my diamonds'. Then comes the self-pity and misery, 'The world doesn't see me and doesn't hear me and they owe me.' Victim.

Comment (JS)

If I asked any homoeopath to guess what remedy this is, Phosphorus would be the last remedy that would come to mind, and that is exactly what makes the proving so accurate. This proving saves us from the one-sided farce that has become the popular essence of Phosphorus – the sympathetic giving, loving side. Of course, that side is there, but it can never exist without the polar opposite, and in this proving, here it is. One can get more of this side from reading the original proving, but Camilla's proving explains it to a higher degree. Phosphorus is a bold type remedy in 'Discontent', and appears in 'Selfishness' and 'Avarice'. When thinking of 'Avarice', remember that in the periodic table, Arsenicum is the daughter of Phosphorus, and that the apple does not fall far from its tree.

This proving picture is further verified when we remember that Phosphorus is the ultimate tubercular remedy. The main idea of tuberculosis is deficiency of oxygen and the resulting constant feeling of lack. Tuberculosis, or consumption, is a disease that eats away our bodies away and leaves us with nothing. When we think of the continual tubercular yearning for more, when we remember the phosphorus fires raging over Hamburg, sucking every molecule of oxygen out of the air, then this proving makes even more sense. Oxygen, the first desire of every human being, has been burnt out of the air and we are left with air hunger and a sense of lack. The proving of Oxygen signifies money, ego and love, which Phosphorus is also screaming out for.

The angle shown in the upper diagram of Figure 14.4 is like a baby just rising from its horizontal state. But it cannot rise further and take care of itself, and so it screams and demands, 'I want, I want, I want', banging its fists on the supermarket floor, 'Me, me, me, you owe me'! This angle is a complementary mirror image to Aluminum's angle. Aluminum has no identity or ego and hence no specific desire, while Phosphorus is all ego and want.

We can notice the opposite and more familiar side of Phosphorus by taking away the negative words in Camilla's proving (see below), and we are left with the simplistic Phosphorus that homoeopaths love to rely on. But God help us from one-sided, two-dimensional essences that are consuming homoeopathy and leaving a great lack in their wake.

Read the bold type, underlined words only (from the proving above): '*This person would not do* **voluntary work** *or* **give for the sake of giving** *or have a* **consciousness of give or receive**, *always a feeling of lack. Such a fundamental lack that I can't give, a miser, the ultimate avarice.*'

The proving of Phosphorus from Allen's *Encyclopedia* presented As If One Person

Delirium, in which the patient got out of bed and was found lying on the floor, screaming frightfully and tossing about. Constant attempts to escape; it was necessary to confine the patient to the bed; Constant frightful screaming and biting, and tearing the pillow with the teeth. Morose and indolent. Inconsolable grief, with weeping and crying, Moaning and groaning, Cried loudly in bursts. Extremely discontented. Discontented and irresolute. My wants were numerous and varied.[7]

Finally it is interesting to note the relationship of the Phosphorus proving and of its parent element Nitrogen. Both represent boundaries or lack of boundaries. Nitrogen relates to the expansion and contraction of boundaries, while Phosphorus has porous boundaries.

Relevant rubrics (*The Complete Repertory*)[5]

Anger children in, with atrophy

Anger, temper tantrums

Anguish, respiratory complaints in

Anxiety, no rest night and day, prevents one from lying down

Avarice

Clinging of children, always take hand of mother, grasps at bystanders

Desires full of, refused when offered

Fear, suffocation

Selfish

Sulphur, Element 16

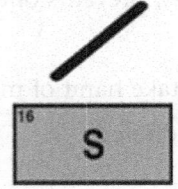

Figure 14.11 *Sulphur*

Sulphur

In the beginning
Was the beginning
Before the beginning
Beginning began
Inventor mutating
Creator creating
Creator created
It's all in a line

Wake up early
Bowels burst
Follow me
Always first
Instigating
Clear the way
I can arrive
But never stay

My fire burns
But not my bush
Nothing to me
Only push
Forward, forward
Just one way
At the end
Begin again

First Meditation Proving

(Bold type JS)

(After two seconds.)

Straight away, it is making me cry, straight away!

(Crying, sobbing, sighing for few minutes.)

Kind of like a crying but a relief to cry, like 'Weeping ameliorates'; like it helped emotionally.

I don't have any clue what that was about. It was straight away, straight away that I wanted to cry, and I wasn't in a weepy mood before.

(Sighing)

I feel like someone with a heavy burden on my shoulders, like my shoulders are slumping and my spine is curling forward.

I feel my period pain in the lower back.

I feel like someone who is exhausted and worn out.

I just feel like crying.

I feel like someone who says, 'I have no strength left', like a wet rag, like a limpet. Like my whole body has gone all limp, like cooked spaghetti. At the same time, I feel like someone too tired to care, an indifference, someone who has resigned and given up.

I am too tired to live, sad and worn out, no point in anything, absolutely no point. But then at the same time, when I say there is no point, I feel like crying, like self-pity. A huge sadness, like something terrible happened. Someone died and something terrible happened and you're going along and remember and the sadness just washes over you. Crying and sobbing in grief.

(Sobbing and sobbing in grief.)

A kind of sadness and depression that you stay in bed and cry all day and can't get up; can't even take a shower or get dressed.

That's it! Don't want to talk about it anymore.

Exhausted, don't want to talk or see anyone, just want to be left alone.

That's it.

Depression and grief and indifference and wanting to be alone.

I want to go to bed, alone.

Comment (JS)

I was most impressed with the repetition of the words *'straight away'* in this mini proving, because I had long ago worked out that geometrically Sulphur is represented by a straight line with no beginning point.

To give an example from Kent's *Lectures on Materia Medica*:

> Sulphur has cured this consecutive tracing one thing to another as to first cause. It has cured a patient who did nothing but meditate as to what caused this and that and the other thing, finally tracing things back to Divine Providence, and then asking "Who made God?". . . . One woman could never see any handiwork of man without asking who made it. She could never be contented until she found out the man who made it, and then she wanted to know who his father was; she would sit down and wonder who he was, whether he was an Irish man, and so on.[8]

Sulphur is always searching for the beginning. Other examples are hunger before a meal, diarrhea in the morning on waking, or the first remedy to begin chronic treatment with, new inventions etc. Read Kent's *Materia Medica* with this idea in mind and you will find it repeated in many different instances.

The opposition to this straight line is the function of 'must curl up'. So that geometrically we can depict Sulphur as follows:

Sensation: No beginning, must go back in a straight line.

Function: Must curl.

This short proving brings out an unknown emotional side of Sulphur, but it is fascinating to see how true to the original proving this aspect is. We are commonly not aware of this side of Sulphur, due to shallow and prejudiced essences and misconception. This proving corrects the 'modern' erroneous notion that Sulphur is not an emotional remedy and specifically that it has no grief. Note that Sulphur is Black Type in many grief symptoms in *The Complete Repertory* 2016.

The proving of Sulphur from Allen's *Encyclopedia*, presented As if One Person.

> Very great weeping mood. During the nightly cough the boy fell into long weeping, with great physical restlessness. Greatly inclined to weep without cause. Moaning and complaining, with wringing of the hands day and night. Extremely sensitive, and weeping easily on the slightest unpleasantness. Despondent, indifferent. Greatly depressed, hypochondriac and sighing, so that he could not speak a loud word (the first weeks). She does not know what to do with herself on account of internal discouragement. Without any cause, great depression of spirits. Sad, without courage or cause. Sad, discouraged, weary of life. While walking in the open air she suddenly became sad; she was filled with only sad, anxious despondent thoughts, from which she could not free herself, which made

her suspicious, peevish, and lachrymose. During the day, sad, lachrymose; she weeps if one attempts to console her. Frequently during the day she has attacks of melancholy when she feels extremely unhappy, without cause; she wishes to die. In the course of the day, without any cause, very melancholy disposition, discontented with himself and all about him, which made him unfit for any serious occupation, and at the same time very irascible.[9]

Second Meditation Proving (3 weeks later)

(Bold type JS)

*Felt it **straight away**.*

*As if elbows and arm joints **became soft and bendy**.*

My throat feels a bit thick and swollen like a lump.

*All joints feel **soft and not straight, bending**.*

*I want to put my elbows **straight, lock them straight**.*

***My back is curved but I want it to be straight, it keeps bending**.*

I don't feel good.

The light from outside seems very bright.

I want my knees to be straight. **(She is forcibly straightening her knees.)**

My thoughts keep wandering, can't focus.

Feel tired and confused, can't formulate my thoughts; can't keep them together; can't connect with myself enough to give symptoms. Feel it's all just chaos; can't grab a thought.

*I can't focus. **Going round and round** in my head without any direction or **point of focus. Nothing knows where it's supposed to go**.*

Everything a mess in my brain, all floating plasma. Everything floating there and no one knows where it's supposed to go, *totally aimless, no definition. Everything swimming along however they feel like flowing or swimming but without any drive, without anywhere to get to, **without and end point**, without a desire outcome. No goal, just random **floating around sporadically and aimlessly, floating around. Nothing is sharp or focus, all soft or brown, nothing is direct. Nothing is direct in a straight line. Want to get there, everything curly, endless, distracted, pointless. Everything is round and curvy, amoeba, Medusa, aimless floating**.*

Someone with no direction or opinion or drive or motivation.

Thoughts floating, no direction.

Sensation that I have to extend my ankles straight, not bendy. *Went from elbows, from knees to ankles, down . . .*

*In a word – **curved ball**, drugged, half in dream world.*

Feels like Valium, half daze.

A lady I know, a philosophical, religious person, was on Valium for years, or a man I know, who is spaced out just doing pottery. No marketing or pushing himself.

I am out of it completely.

*Image of lady I know on a scooter **driving in straight line** to save her husband shouting, 'I'm coming I'm coming'. A scooter, sea or land, **going fast in a straight line. Very direct in a straight line.***

No energy at all. Whole body in limbo, can't sit up.

(Asked her to sit up. She is sitting up . . .)

Better for sitting upright.

Feel more clear upright.

My focus is back. Much more present.

Feel much better when upright, *a dramatic difference, have direction.*

Comment (JS)
This second mini proving strengthens and clarifies the main idea of the previous mini proving and the original proving. We see the prominent theme of a straight line versus curve.

We might sum it up as: No beginning or end points, must proceed to search for them in a straight line. Direct and straight logic searching in a straight line for a beginning that can never be found. Empty philosophizing – logic with no beginning or base. The opposite function is curving and bending into aimless chaos.

Note that the Sulphur angle in the upper diagram of Figure 14.4 is the mirror and complement to Magnesium. Magnesium is the orphan that had a start but no guidance beyond the beginning. He cannot transcend the childish beginning into adulthood, while Sulphur, the adult, is always searching for a beginning. This teaches us something of the real inner nature of Sulphur. Perhaps the grief indicates a person who had no beginning through death of parents or similar, and hence experiences perpetual grief and no childhood. He is forced to grow up too quickly, but is always searching for his beginnings, allowing straight logic to suppress curved emotions

The following symptom from the original proving of Sulphur might indicate someone of this disposition:

> Vexatious and morbid ideas of the past arise from the most indifferent thoughts, and from every occurrence in life, which continue to be united with new vexations, so that she cannot free herself from them, together with a courageous mood which is ready for great resolution.[9]

Of course, there will be something of Magnesium in Sulphur and vice versa.

Chlorine, Element 17

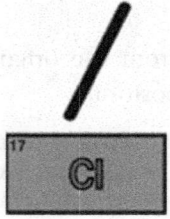

Figure 14.12 *Chlorine*

Chlorum

Contraction
Glottis shoved down my throat
Fat lumpy thyroid
Choking my breath
Adam!
Kindly remove your apple
From my throat.

I feel this is going deep, deep, deep. Deep into my stomach.

(She is making a deep echoing sound *Hhaaaa*. Again, mouthing *Hoooooo* in a deep echoing way.)

Deep, deep into the stomach.

(Sighing.)

Ow ow ow (moaning), *pain in my coccyx, the tip of my tail bone suddenly hurting, sharp pain. That is exactly where it went. Root Chakra. Totally to my coccyx, also genitals.*

(Moaning) *Haaaaa* (in a deep voice).

This is like when I gave birth, the same sound coming from me as I made during birth, deep, deep. (Groans) *AHHHH.* (I can verify these were the same sounds she made during birth, and at no other time – JS)

I might give birth. Oh God.

Now the same pain in my finger, a sharp pain. Ow!!!!

Sharp, cutting pains.

Now I feel my hip.

(Doing a rocking motion like when giving birth.) *This has activated my whole pelvis.*

Feel I need to rock and move, just like when I was in labour, exactly like labour. Wow, I must have stored some stuff there, something left over.

(She is squatting and leaning over a low table, like a woman in labour.)

Wow, I didn't know I had all that stuff there. I think I've released it!

(Now squatting on the floor.)

(She is standing and moving her hips in circular motion.)

Wow. I just realize I've been like a stiff plank. I think I stored a lot from that labor, hormones, maybe trauma?

(She is standing and moving her hips in circular motion.)

I feel a lot of energy in my pelvis and root chakra and I need to move it, belly dance. I can't believe I've been storing this for 18 years! It took me back to my 18-year-old son's birth.

(She is moving around in a flexible way, rotating her pelvis, bending double, shaking arms as if enjoying a new freedom of motion.)

It feels fantastic. It feels as if suddenly my whole pelvis and lower back can move. Oh my God, this feels so good!

(She is doing yoga and birth positions, moving around on the floor and rocking to and fro.)

My whole pelvis has become unstuck and is opening up.

(Dancing around on the floor.) *Oh wow, wow, wow. I feel so much energy surging though my body. Yay!*

I bet you most women have this. And I had the easiest births, only five hours.

When I press into my abdomen, my uterus feels tender, painful.

(Doing calf stretches and rotations and flexing exercise, rocking pelvis from side to side with a sense of joy and release.) *I feel SO good!*

It is clearly all my pelvis, the rest not involved at all (dancing).

Give this to every woman who ever gave birth! Amazing, it hit the tip of my tailbone, where every woman gets damaged when giving birth. How can they not, it's in the way!

WOW! Awesome.

(She is walking around the room, waggling her bum from side to side.) *I feel my posture is different, straighter and taller.*

You know the sexy walk women do. Well after a few kids it goes away. It's just come back. Like all my pelvic ligaments are suddenly loose and floatable. (Wagging bum from side to side.) *This must have released the birth hormones (Relaxin, oxyctocin??). I think it just released all my hormones, like when about to give birth. After you give birth, it's supposed to tighten up naturally, but I think hardly anyone does it right. You tighten too much, remain in pain and trauma, don't come together right, something is stored.*

Sensation of leucorrhoea, as if uterus clearing out.

(Sitting on floor and touching toes.) *Wow, I can go much further than I usually can after an hour of yoga!*

I just feel fabulous! Such satisfaction in stretching.

I feel like this woman we know who walks with a hip wag, always strutting her stuff. She just came into my head. Always strutting her stuff, wiggling her bum when she walks, free, no constrictions, just liberty. Do what you want, don't care about anyone. Older people are her constriction and limiting factor, but she just does what she wants. The point in life when you are still so narcissistic, like a two-year-old, where your own self is all you see. You don't even know or see other people. The liberty is in the fact that others are not even a consideration. Absolute self-centeredness. Life is so simple when you're not considering other people. Others don't matter.

(After learning the remedy is Chlorine, element 17.)

That's it, a 17-year-old! Do what you want!

I feel like 17 is significant, like someone who is 17. No responsibilities, just strutting your stuff. Wiggling your bum, wearing tiny shorts, not cleaning up after yourself, not helping, just fantastically self-absorbed and only interested in yourself, not seeing others. Freedom, don't care, don't even think it's an issue, or that there is an issue. Lovely feeling of doing what you want, being free, stretching . . . no responsibilities. I think I'll go and stretch or exercise, someone else can cook. I feel tall and lean and hot. I think I'll go and put on makeup. How wonderful to be like this. Simply narcissistic, only I matter. I feel so free. All the tightness in my pelvis is releasing, going . . . it's wonderful. I think I'll stretch some more. Heaven. I will always strut my stuff from now on. What a relief, a release. It all got so tight after I gave birth for the first time.

Something matures in you after you give birth. Suddenly you have to care for others all the time. You don't strut your stuff because you might get pregnant again! In pregnancy you expand in a way you never thought possible and then you push a human being out of your vagina. Constriction and expansion. After that, it's all responsibility, thinking of other people, being there for others. You don't have a mama to pick up clothes for you; you are the mama. This is the natural state of a 17-year-old. It's right to be free and no responsibility and wiggle your ass at 17, a God-given state, a birthright. But not at 33.

Connected to sexuality. Like when I was 17 and left home. Before that my mum constricted me so much, curfews, I was not allowed to do this and not allowed to do that. The idea was that if they don't constrict me I will strut my stuff and have affairs and get pregnant – not good from their point of view. When I left home I was free to do what I wanted selfishly. Like this!

(JS asked, What if you combine this with Chlorum–Natrum muriaticum?)

Oh my God! Fuck! Disaster! Just pain. A loss of your identity, of who you are. Of Natrum combined with selfish, strut your stuff – they don't suit at all! Unsuitable lovers!

Comment (JS)
This is an under-proved remedy, so there is not much to compare to. The proving surprised me because I was expecting it to be a nasty experience as in the gas poisonings and the materia medica, but as usual, Camilla brings out the opposite, this time the positive side.

The main theme in the Chlorine materia medica is constriction, usually of throat and respiratory organs. It is also listed as having stiffness. In this proving we get the opposite idea of release from tightness and restriction on freedom.

This proving represents another step in the journey of self-realization and actualization of a teenager that begins with Natrum and culminates in Argon. Just as in its parent element Fluorine[i], Chlorum's main power is constriction, and as we see here, the removal of constrictions.

Because chlorine is so reactive, it never occurs freely in nature. The small proving in our materia medica is not pure chlorine.

Psychological Themes: Erotic, Sexuality, Altruism (opposite).

Related rubrics (*The Complete Repertory*)[5]
Mind, Attached, mother to

Mind, Boisterous, out-going

Mind, Comfort, sensation of

Generals, Tendons

Generals, Relaxation

Generals, Relaxation, Muscles

Generals, Stiffness, rigidity

Female, Leucorrhoea

---

[i] See: Fluorine. In: Sherr J. *The Dynamic Materia Medica of Noble Gases: Neon.* Glasgow: Saltire Books, 2016.

Muriaticum-natronatum

She asked for a happy poem
And I faltered,
Not knowing where
Or how
To clutch
The dancing days of spring
To my autumn heart
Or conjure from a world unknown
Balloons of floating yellow red
Of hollow birthday merriment
Adorned by prancing major scales.

Then fathoming familiar depths
Of rocky sea-beds deep below
From which my song does cry to rise
And burst upon this bubbling mind
Extracting pleasure
Forged in pain
Far sweeter
Then the tinkling glitter
Of happiness.

Argon

Rays of sun glitter the
waters of enchanted childhood,
Fairy footsteps dancing
mermaids, pixie dust
spermatozoa gaily swimming
upstream; unobstructed, carefree, exploring
new dimensions of blossoming adulthood, forbidden
thoughts wagging tales of puppy
love speckled with a hidden kiss
and grope, fresh green saplings sprouting
innocently skywards as otters roll play
beach parties;
time
cannot touch us now
bundled in our magic.
Eternal youth.

Three

Three forces
Make new life
Mother's egg, father's sperm
and
God's holy touch.
In the warm darkness
I wait
For waters to burst
Earth to rise
The tree of life to grow.

Sodium preserves the seed
Magnesium lends a life,
Alum cut from mother
By a surgeon's knife,
Silica will penetrate
From cervix into air
Phos and Sulph ignite the flame
Chlor puts boundaries there
Until the child will blossom
Together with its tree;
Childhood sweet
Summer fruits
Own identity.

References

1 Kent JT. Alumina. *Lectures on Homeopathic Materia Medica*. Available online at: http://homeoint.org/books3/kentmm/alm.htm

2 Vermeulen F. Alumina. In: *Ultimate Prisma Collection. Synoptic Reference – 1*. Glasgow: Saltire Books, 2015. pp95–96.

3 Moore PB, Edwardson JA, Farrier IN *et al.* Gastrointestinal absorption of aluminum is increased in Down's syndrome. *Biol Psychiatry*. 1997 Feb 15; 41(4):488–92. Abstract available online at: https://www.ncbi.nlm.nih.gov/pubmed/9034543

4 Dialysis dementia. Merriam-Webster Medical Dictionary. Available online at: https://www.merriam-webster.com/medical/dialysis%20dementia

5 Van Zandvoort R, ed. *The Complete Repertory* in RADAR 10 Archibel Homeopathic Software, 2015.

6 Kent JT. Silica. *Lectures on Homeopathic Materia Medica*. Available online at: http://homeoint.org/books3/kentmm/sil.htm

7 Allen TF. P'hosphorus. *Pure Materia Medica*. In: *Encyclopedia Homeopathica*. Archibel Software.

8 Kent JT. Sulphur. *Lectures on Homeopathic Materia Medica*. Available online at: http://homeoint.org/books3/kentmm/sul.htm

9 Allen TF. Sulphur. *Pure Materia Medica*. In: *Encyclopedia Homeopathica*. Archibel Software.

15

ARGON MM ANALOGY, BIOLOGY, COSMOLOGY

A homoeopath must learn to weave a web of meaning.
J Sherr

Biblical parallels

The following are interpretations of the correspondences between the periodic table, the noble gas provings, the physical and temporal dimensions, the seven days of creation and other biblical stories from the Book of Genesis. These comparisons are made throughout the 'Noble Gas' series in order to shed light on all these aspects so as to deepen our overall understanding and perception. The correspondences are remarkable, each being a mirror image of the great universal plan as it unfolds. These connections are certainly one of the 'Biblical codes'.

So far we have seen that each day of creation parallels a period in the periodic table and culminates with the words 'It was good,' which corresponds to the relative noble gas. Now we will widen the perspective.

First portion: 'Genesis'

The original Hebrew bible is divided into portions, rather than chapters, which are a 13th century addition. Each portion has a name. The first portion of Genesis is named 'Genesis' and includes the story of creation, followed by the story of the Garden of Eden and the history of the first people and their deeds on earth. This portion corresponds to the first period, Hydrogen and Helium, representing the world of primary creative power, heavenly potential and its first terrestrial manifestation.[i] Specifically,

---

[i] See discussion in Sherr J. *The Noble Gases. Helium including an introduction to the Noble Gases*. Glasgow: Saltire Books, 2013.

Hydrogen relates to the big bang, 'Let there be light' and the seven days of creation, while Helium to the story of Adam and Eve and their first descendants. This first period also represents the first physical dimension, that of a line. A line stretches between two points, a binary 'this or that'. This first dimension is reflected in Helium's simple binary dilemma of 'to be or not to be'. Similarly, we see that the outcome of the creation days is also one-dimensional and binary: Light and dark, sky and water, earth and land, sun and moon, fish and bird, female and male, good and bad. There are no shades of human complexity. All is simple.

Second portion: 'Noah'

The second portion is called 'Noah', telling the story of the great flood. It corresponds to the second day of creation, the noble gas Neon and the second physical dimension of surface. The proving of Neon mentions both the second day and the story of Noah.[i] On the second day the waters separate in two surfaces- sky and sea. In the Noah story, after the great flood there is water everywhere. Water always finds its own level, hence it is a flat surface, and represents the second dimension. A surface can be defined by three points; Noah bears three sons.

Ten generations separate Adam and Noah, just as Hydrogen is element number 1 and Neon is number 10. The name Noah means 'rest' or 'comfort', symbolizing the tranquil noble gases.

Noah brings the animals into the ark, two by two, reminding us of the two-dimensionality of this story. The emotional aspects of this story are two-dimensional and reflect Neon's childish and superficial personality. The story is a children's favorite. Noah, a noble and righteous person, is not elaborated upon; he has a two-dimensional and simple personality. The Bible states that he is virtuous, but it is in a naïve sort of way, typical of Neon. In this portion even God appears two-dimensional (from our 'flat' point of view). At first he is angry with Noah, but later repents and promises never to flood the earth again, a pledge he seals with a Neon rainbow in the sky. The story ends with Noah getting drunk, a reminder of Neon's addictive side. Neon, Noah, Day Two and two-dimensional surface form a meaningful group.

As the flood waters recede, dry land appears. While the 'water-earth' separation relates to Day Three of creation (first half), we have already

---

[i] See discussion in Sherr J. *Dynamic Materia Medica of the Noble Gases: Neon.* Glasgow: Saltire Books, 2016, p186.

established that this actually is the completion of the 'water work' project from Day Two and belongs to Day Two. The water project ends with the words '*It was good*', the Biblical code for a noble gas, in this case Neon, and we now move down to the third period and the beginning of the third physical dimension of 'sphere,' for which we will need height. The separation of earth and water reminds us of Alumina and the ability of clay pots, pans and puddles to separate earth and water.

Third portion: 'Go Forth'[i]

We move on to the third Biblical portion, the third day, the third period and the third dimension.

Three generations after Noah, his descendants attempt to penetrate into the third dimension by building the tower of Babel, a vertical challenge to God. When they fail, as the tower collapses, they are scattered throughout the world and are made to speak different languages. As a consequence, humanity suffers an inability to communicate (Natrium) and confusion of identity (Alumina). 'Babel' literally means confusion.

In the second half of the third day and of the third period, Silica, Phosphorus and Sulphur generate trees that sprout skywards and produce fruit, unfolding the third dimension. As this dimension expands, the constricted surface of the second dimension opens its passageways, resulting in free-flowing motion. The corresponding third portion of Genesis is literally called 'Go forth', and tells tales of many travels and the crossing great rivers. Avram (later Avraham or Abraham) is told to walk over 1500 km to the Promised Land. Because Avram has crossed the great rivers, the Praat and the Jordan, he is named a Hebrew – meaning 'he who has crossed the water'. As such, Avram is like the amphibians of Argon, easily navigating over earth and water. He then travels to Egypt and back, where he wanders freely throughout the Promised Land of Canaan and as far north as Damascus.

This biblical story portrays a three-dimensional emotional complexity, involving love triangles. One of the triangles comprises Avram, his stunningly beautiful wife Saray (later renamed Sarah) and a love-struck Pharaoh who steals her. This is followed by another love triangle, this time involving Avram, Saray and her maid servant Hagar. The competition between the two women concerns fertility, a prominent issue in this portion. The words sperm or seed, third day and Argon issues, are mentioned often.

---

[i] The Hebrew words לֶךְ-לְךָ ('*Lech, lecha*') translate literally as 'You will walk', or 'Go walk'.

Avram splits from his nephew Lot, who goes left to the wet fertile land, while Avram turns to the sea, a reminder of Day Three separation. God tells Avram to '*Arise*, walk through the land in the *length* of it and in the *breadth* of it; for unto thee will I give it', a sentence including all three dimensions. In true Argon manner, Avram and Saray do not come of age or become fertile until they are in their 90's, when God renames them Abraham and Sarah, signifying their spiritual ripeness. She falls pregnant, the perfect conclusion to the third period. It seems that their first 90 years were but an extended childhood leading to late maturity. Their relationship with God also matures, going beyond the simple concepts of good and bad into a complex set of negotiations and covenants.

Fourth portion: 'And He Appeared'

Here the billion-dollar existential question must arise, having been ignored and mis-explained for so long. Why does everyone up to this biblical time live until they are nine hundred years old, and continue to have children at well over one hundred years? The answer lies in Krypton, which represents the fourth dimension of time and the fourth day of creation, in which moon and sun and stars spin cycles. Speaking of stars, in the corresponding fourth portion of Genesis, aliens will arrive on earth through stargates, carrying lasers and nuclear weapons. Salt will freeze time; watch this space. . . .

Biology

The genetics of incarnation

In the previous books of this series the first two nobles, Helium and Neon, were compared to the process of meiosis. Helium correlated to telophase I, the first stage of meiosis, in which the parent cell divides into two daughter cells, and Neon to the second stage, telophase II, where each daughter cell splits into two haploid gametes containing half as many chromosomes as the original cell.

The end result of this process is a single haploid, or half-cell, sperm or ovum, waiting expectantly for its other half, its soul 'ga-mate'. At first the gametes are tranquil but as the time of meeting grows nearer they begin to itch with desire. Certainly the ovum is reminiscent of the cosmic egg waiting to be breached. There are several references to ova in the Neon proving.

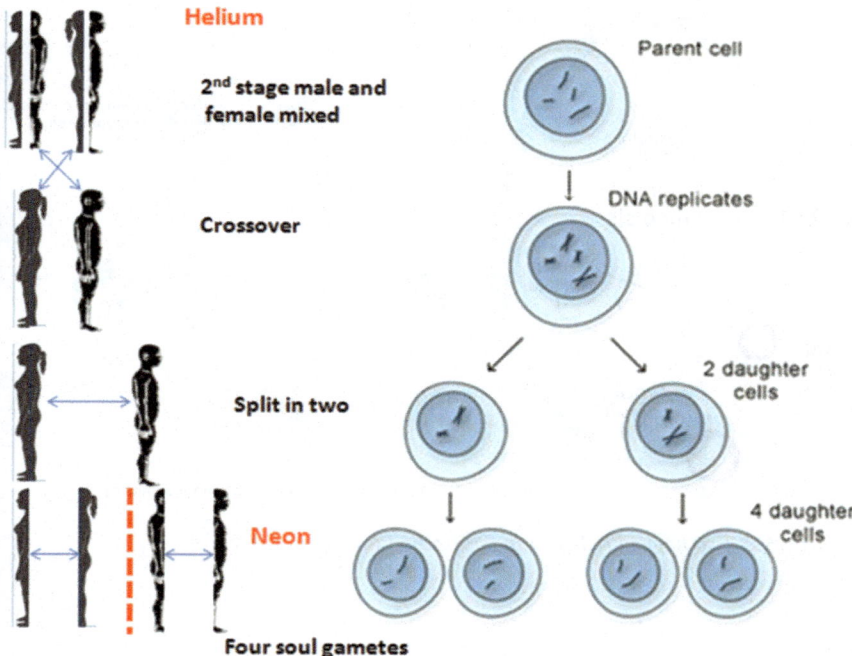

Figure 15.1 Telophases I and II

I felt like I was an unfertilised egg, an ovum, very peaceful. (Neon)

When a woman is born, her ova are ready and present. Each ovum must patiently wait her turn in the ovary tower, until one day in the distant future a gallant knight, riding a white horse with a swishing tail, will penetrate her membrane. Sperm, seed and fertilization appear in the third day story. If all goes well, two haploid cells will unite cells into a single diploid cell in the sacred marriage of a zygote-the "Argon moment". Two strands of DNA, one half from mother and one half from father, will combine as one in a spiral dance to form the beginning of life. The Argon proving reflects this process:

Cells only split when they're horizontal.

I was only saying half of the true time or quantity. Things were half price or two for one.

In the dance, it's only possible at that angle if the support is mutual. The dance formed an alliance.

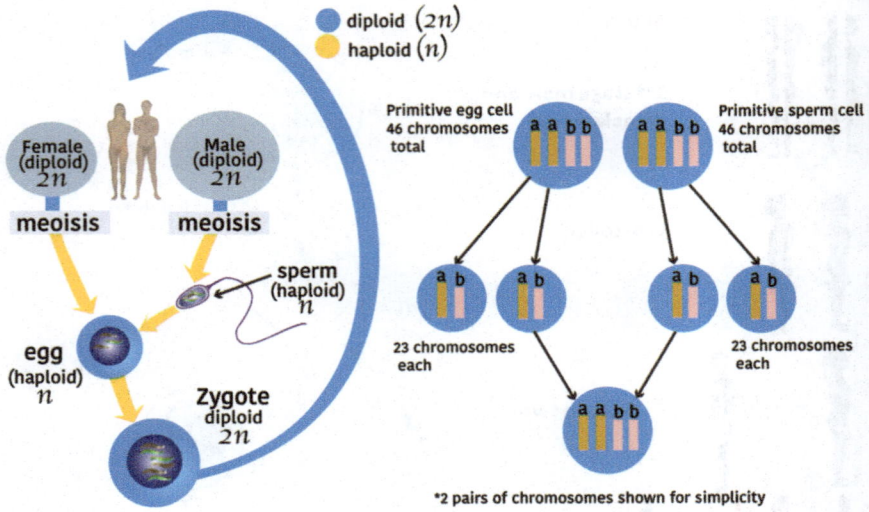

Figure 15.2 Two haploid cells join in fertilization to form a zygote

DNA

In the *Helium* and *Neon* books, protein synthesis is discussed.[i] Once a new cell is formed, it must create protein. The instructions for protein production are transferred from DNA, residing in the cell nucleus, to the cell cytoplasm by means of RNA. Amino acids are constructed according to these directions. The whole process involves the steps known as transcription and translation.

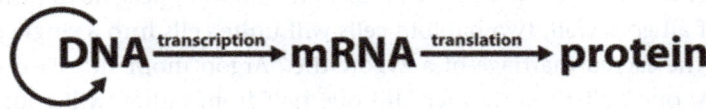

Figure 15.3 DNA replication, transcription and translation

Before transcription, the DNA double helix must first replicate itself by unzipping its two strands and duplicating them to become four. Helium is analogous to DNA replication. The transcription stage follows, in which the duplicated strands are unzipped again into mirror images of each other and are copied onto messenger RNA (mRNA). DNA has two strands arranged in a double helix, while mRNA consists of a single strand, which is transported

---

[i] See Chapter 9 in Sherr, *Helium* and Chapter 16 in Sherr, *Neon*.

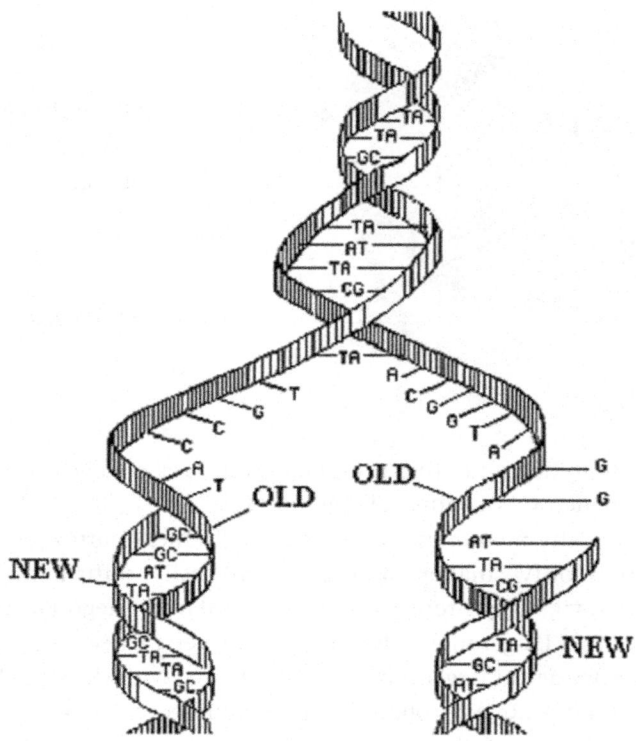

Figure 15.4 DNA transcription phase

out of the nucleus to the cytoplasm. The remaining DNA then zips up behind it. Neon corresponds to the transcription phase.

We were all trying each other's clothes/costumes on. JS said I owed him lots of money and to check my records. He said I could pay him just half of what was owed. I then said, 'No, I will double it', i.e. I would pay double what I owed. Then I was travelling and sat at the rear end, on a seat which had half a seat beside it. The two back seats were one-and-a half each, while those in front were just normal.

The next stage of the process is translation. The messenger RNA migrates out of the nucleus and into the cytoplasm, passing through pores in the nuclear membrane. The nuclear membrane completely encloses the nucleus and separates the cell's genetic material from the surrounding cytoplasm. It serves as a barrier to prevent large molecules from diffusing freely between the nucleoplasm and the cytoplasm. The transportation of mRNA is further controlled by complex 'export mechanisms', which do not allow

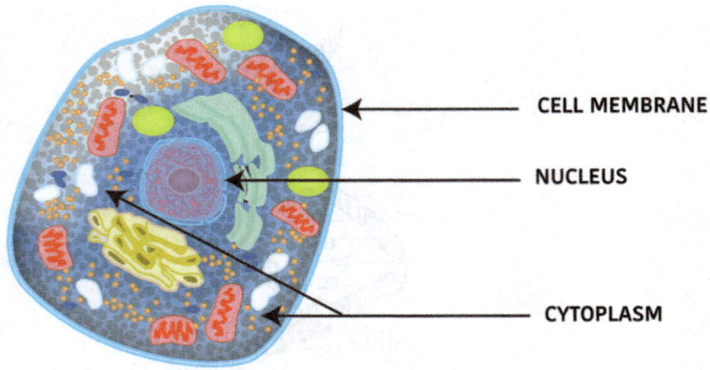

Figure 15.5 Cell

immature pre-mRNA and other undesirables such as nucleic acids and large proteins to penetrate out through the pores.

The gaps in the membrane or pores are extremely narrow, about 9 nm wide, so that only smaller molecules can easily diffuse through the membrane. Navigating through these pores is akin to 'negotiating through a 3-D labyrinth'.[1] Larger molecules cannot transverse these narrow passages. The blocked passage of larger molecules, compared with the straightforward transportation of mRNA through the membrane pores, is analogous to the obstructed versus free-flowing motion seen in Argon. Only 'mature' mRNA molecules can pass the barrier.

Thought we were closer to side of road, like the road was narrower and closing in.

Travel again easy today and what could have turned out to be very diffi-cult crossing was in fact **plain sailing**.

The passage from inner nucleoplasm to outer cytoplasm can also be compared to life's early passage from sea to land.

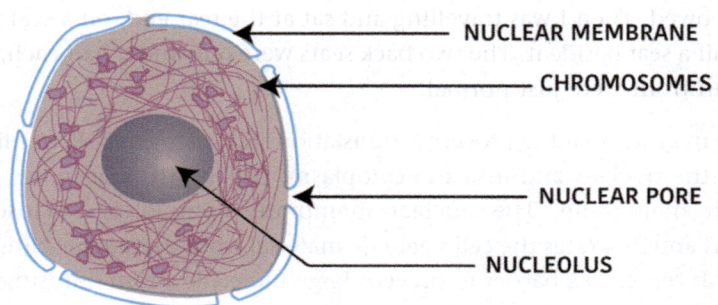

Figure 15.6 Cell with nuclear pores in membrane

Tetractys

The tetractys is an ancient symbol of sacred geometry that held much significance among the Pythagoreans and Cabbalists. Pythagoras, the ancient Greek philosopher and mathematician, regarded it as a symbol of the arithmetic, geometric and musical ratios upon which the universe is built.

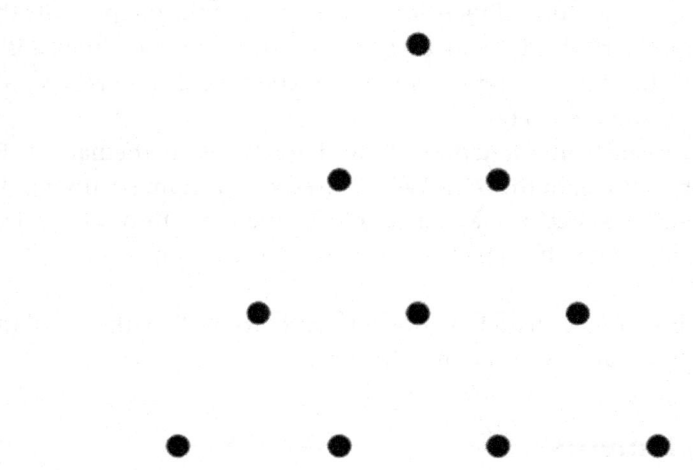

Figure 15.7 Tetractys

This prayer of the Pythagoreans shows the importance of the Tetractys:

Bless us, divine number, thou who generated gods and men! O holy, holy Tetractys, thou that containest the root and source of the eternally flowing creation! For the divine number begins with the profound, pure unity until it comes to the holy four; then it begets the mother of all, the all-comprising, all-bounding, the first-born, the never-swerving, the never-tiring holy ten, the keyholder of all.[2]

The tetractys is a triangle composed of ten points arranged in four rows: one, two, three, and four points in each row, similar to the way pins are arranged in a bowling lane.

For Pythagoras the lines of the tetractys hold these meanings:[3]

The first row is made of a single point representing zero-dimensions, the divine dimension from which everything is created. It is usually associated with the virtue of wisdom.

The second row symbolizes one-dimension (a line connecting two points) and 'Neikos' or Strife. Strife, or argument, is the power of division and is often associated with the virtues of movement and impulse.

The third row signifies two-dimensions (a plane defined by a triangle of three points), an image of harmony and mental balance.

The fourth row depicts three-dimensions (a tetrahedron defined by four points). The four points indicate the four elements of the ancient world: earth, air, fire and water.

Comparing this interpretation to our study of the noble gases, we see that the first singularity represents the pre-Hydrogen state before the Big Bang. The second row is the single dimension of Helium, the third represents the two-dimensional surface of Neon and the fourth the three-dimensional Argon. It is in the third period of Argon that the four elements, fire, air, earth and water, are completed.

The Pythagoreans' interpretation of the tetractys is mathematical. By contrast, Cabbalists regard the tetractys as a mystical diagram signifying the way the universe is structured, and a parallel to the ten seffirot of the Tree of Life. They also link the tetractys with the Tetragrammaton, the holy name of God.

The "one into four" model of the tetractys fits well with the soul's division into four parts, as elaborated in *Helium*.

The four elements

The four elements, fire, air, earth and water, are a simple map of nature, one that has proved useful as a tool for understanding materia medica and patients. On the first day and the first period, God creates light or **Fire**, the fusion of hydrogen into helium. On the second day and period, **Air** appears as oxygen, followed by **Water**, the combination of hydrogen and oxygen. On the third day and period the waters separate to expose the **Earth**, containing elements such as magnesium, alumina, sulphur and silica. As the period progresses, the four elements combine to grow vegetation.

In the human body the four elements correspond to the primary organs: heart (fire), lungs (air), kidney (water) and colon (earth). The liver resides in the middle, its important functions similar to that of a tree, synthesising, detoxifying and producing biochemicals. Each of the four elements relates to the organic molecules: hydrogen, nitrogen, oxygen and carbon, which is the central element that holds the organic world together with its four bonding arms (Figure 15.8).

In accordance with the figure above, argon should be aligned with the vertical line of fire and air, since argon can take the place of oxygen and be an asphyxiant. By replacing oxygen, which is a factor in aging, argon acts as a preservative or anti-oxidant. It defers aging in the way argon gas

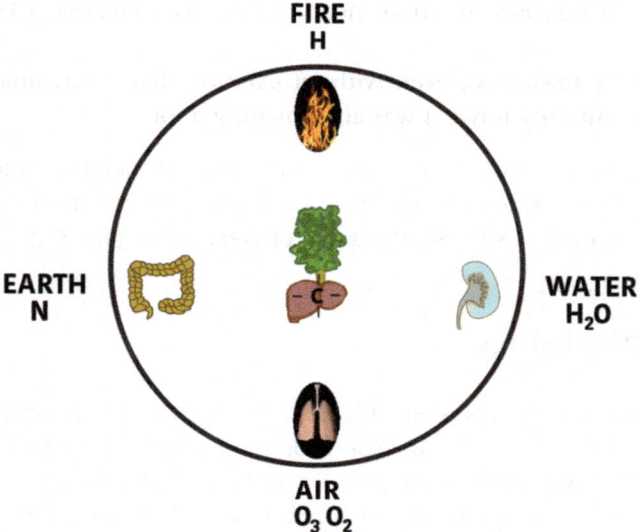

Figure 15.8 Circle of four elements and organic molecules

preserves the filament in a light bulb. Argon, the remedy, has a number of respiratory problems.

Dream, that my husband died. We put him in a plastic bag and tied it at the bottom so that he was completely sealed in the bag.

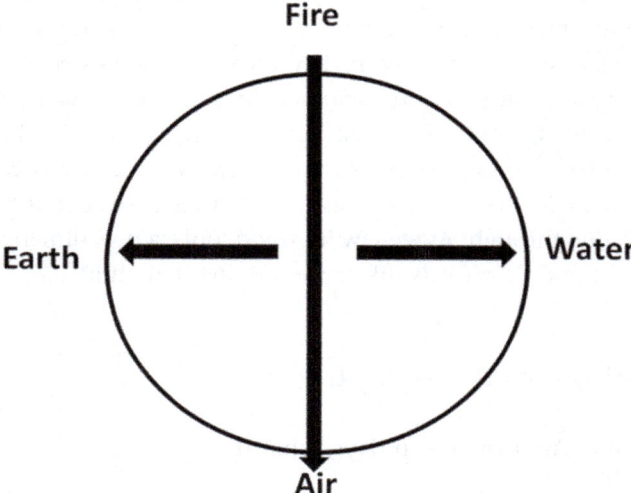

Figure 15.9 Fire-Air axis splits Earth and Water

Feeling of tightness in chest, need to take deep breaths, a kind of 'air hunger'.

I was very breathless, even without exertion; like I was unable to get enough air into my lungs. I was also yawning a lot.

By uniting fire and air, the male and female principles, Argon creates new life. But the Argon axis of Fire – Air also splits Earth from Water, intellect from emotion, as in the third day of creation (Figure 15.9).

Alchemical stage

In the transformative process of alchemy the third step is Separation.[4] In this stage filtration isolates the solid components that have been dissolved into liquid in the previous step of Dissolution. Any unworthy or impure materials are removed from the solution and discarded. The process of Separation is referred to as 'Terrae', meaning 'Of the Earth', since pure essences are released from the unwanted sediments. In the ancient Arcanum Experiment, the compound sodium carbonate, is associated with Separation because it settles out of water and appears as white soda ash on dry lakebeds. The alchemists referred to this compound as Natron. Another symbol of this alchemical stage is the formation of land masses and islands by the powerful forces of Air, Water, Earth, and Fire. The operation of Separation fits well with the third period, which contains sodium (Na), and to the third day of creation, the drying of the seas.

Physiologically, Separation is achieved by following and controlling the breath to give birth to new energy. Psychologically, Separation is seen as a conscious process in which we review formerly suppressed material and decide what to discard so as to refine our personalities. What is discarded may be prejudices, emotional blockages, and feelings we are ashamed of or were taught to hide away. The course of Separation releases the blocked energy by breaking down learned restrictions that obstruct our true nature, so we can shine through. As we saw in Argon, once a new dimension opens, we can let go and flow freely, like an unadulterated child.

Numerology and word puzzles

90 + 18 = 108. After the seven days, what then?

This is a puzzling expression from the proving. Here is my understanding of it:

18, the atomic number of Argon, signifies the tree of life in Hebrew. 90 in Hebrew signifies the righteous one, Tsadik, the upright person who stands at 90 degrees to the earth.

The combination of the two, tree of life and upright person gives 108, which is considered to be a sacred number in many traditions, as well as mathematically significant. Of course, 108 is the same as 18, only with a significant 'nothing' added in between.

Here is another puzzle:

Waking dream: of being really happy and asked whether it was happy with an 'i' or a 'y'. I was told if I was happy with an 'i' i.e. 'hapi', he helped resurrect Osiris by suckling him. Hapy with a 'y' was one of Horus's, who was one of Osiris's sons. This son was in charge of the jar with the lungs in it. I was told it was an honour for Man to fall into the Nile and be eaten by a crocodile. I was told crocodiles are good because they eat rough (both not smooth and not good quality) fish, and that the sun energy was to warm and dry me out.

There are many direct references to Argon themes of water, earth, fertility and the growth of plants in this dream. Hapy or Hapi, depicted as having large breasts, is the god of the annual flooding of the Nile, which deposits fertile soil on the riverbanks. Hap, which may mean 'Nile', was a son of Horus and protector of the lungs. He was also a sign of the North, which is the delta area (water, silt, fertile land) of Egypt. Osiris was god of underworld and death and rebirth inherent in the agricultural cycle of planting and harvesting grain. The Crocodile god was a water god, who came out of the river to its banks and laid its eggs on land, bringing new life. It was considered an honor by the cult that worshiped the Crocodile god for man to fall into the Nile and be eaten by a crocodile.

Here is another for you to dwell on. Whatever the case, things are not what they used to be:

343 degrees. The 17,18, is not quite what we see now, it's what we used to see. Whatever this substance is it sees the heavens differently than what we see now, so the angle of the milky way and the big dipper is different to what we see now. The Mayans describe the milky way as a tree in water, but where the roots are is the mouth of the crocodile.

In the last sentence we see the two dimensional crocodile sprouting the three dimensional tree.

Throat Chakra

So far in studying the noble gases we have seen the correspondence of Helium to the spiritual crown chakra and Neon to the intellectual brow chakra. This theme continues with Argon, which relates to the throat chakra, governing speech, expression and communication, including both hearing and sound.

Feels like my jaw is firmly shut.

Felt like my mouth was open a lot – open-mouthed. Desire to communicate, even though under water.

Felt like I was listening very intensely.

Felt like there was either a deafness or a constant listening out.

The more intensely I listened, the less likely I was to hear it.

You've got the light, but you haven't heard the sound.

Fascination with the word INVOICE. Something to do with payment. Inner voice.

Anxiety about not being able to hear if I was called.

Peter Pan

Every noble gas reflects at least one superhero. Peter Pan, the title character of a J.M Barrie's popular play and book, is the superhero for Argon. The proving had many references to elements of this classic story, such as flying, shadows, fairies, crocodiles, mermaids and lost boys. This observation has been confirmed clinically.

Also known as 'The Boy Who Wouldn't Grow Up', Peter Pan is eternally youthful, daring and playful, and he can fly. Initially he loses his shadow, thus joining the two-dimensional world of the three children he has befriended (surface has no shadow). Wendy, the eldest sister of the children, quickly sews Peter's shadow on him again, and all the children graduate into a three-dimensional youth. A bit of magic dust and now the kids can fly too. Time plays no part in Peter's world. Living in Never Never Land he enjoys an eternal, carefree adolescence, playing with lost boys, mermaids and fairies while fighting off pirates and crocodiles. Captain Hook, in contrast, represents the somber world of adulthood, where the clock is always ticking; the fourth dimension beckons.

Given the many ways in which Peter Pan echoes Argon, it is interesting to examine the life of Peter's creator, J.M. Barrie. Significantly, Barrie's mother was orphaned when she was eight years old and had to take on the household responsibilities, bringing her childhood to an abrupt and early end. Barrie was the ninth child of ten. He was a small child and remained short as an adult. When he was six years old, his brother David, who was fourteen, died. His mother was devastated, and Barrie tried to fill David's place by acting like him, even wearing his older brother's clothes and whistling in a similar way to him. Barrie's mother found comfort in the fact that her dead son would remain a boy forever, never able to grow up and leave her. It has been speculated that this trauma induced psychogenic dwarfism, and was responsible for Barrie's short stature and apparently asexual adulthood.

Barrie was inspired to name his motherly character, Wendy, from his friendship with a little girl, Margaret, who died when she was six years old. She had nicknamed Barrie, 'my friendy', but because of a speech defect, she pronounced it, 'fwendy'. We see that many of Peter Pan's and Barrie's life themes relate to premature deaths that freeze childhood.

Part of Barrie's story is featured in the semi-biographical movie *'Finding Neverland'*. Prior to writing his famous play, Barrie has a platonic relationship with a widow, Silvia Davies, who has young sons. Barrie, married but childless, becomes a surrogate father to them and inspires them with happy, carefree and lively childhood antics. He later incorporated these boys into his play, *'The boy who never grew old'*, focusing on one child, Peter, who is troubled. Of course, time wins in the end when Silvia, who is sick with cancer, is plucked from their lives, leaving the Davies boys orphaned. In real life, Barrie became their guardian.

King David

King David is the biblical hero for Argon. Described as youthful and vital, full of mischief and tricks, he retains his teenager character through much of his life. Like Peter Pan with Captain Hook, King David is always fighting and evading the serious and depressed King Saul (Saul was extremely tall, a somber adult figure). Even as an adult, King David is prone to dancing in the streets, and he dies with a teenage girl in his bed.

Because of his youthful folly and indiscretions, King David is not permitted to build the Jewish Temple in Jerusalem. This is left to his son, King Solomon, who 'being the wisest man' cracks the cryptic code of knowledge. The Temple contained many secrets codes, typical of Krypton.

192 The Noble Gases – Argon

Cinema and entertainment

> Indeed, the best coming-of-age movies are almost always fish-out-of-water films; the water is our youth, and coming of age is how we acclimate ourselves to it.[5]
>
> Dustin Rowles

Audiences love Argon films, which is not surprising given that the magic of adolescence is so attractive. Argon's youthful themes feature so frequently in movies that one might even suspect that Hollywood is a factory of childish dreams. One of the numerous productions of *Peter Pan* is the movie '*Hook*' starring Robin Williams as an ageing Peter Pan. Williams himself was theatrically an Argon-like eternal child. Many of his movies, such as '*Good Morning Vietnam*' '*The Fisher King*' or '*Dead Poets' Society*', were about youthful adults who instill playful innocence and humour into the serious world of adulthood. In these movies there is a continuous clash between two forces, many characters who succumb to time and one that refuses to do so. Williams also brushes closely with Krypton by featuring in the movie '*The Timekeeper*', and desiring to play The Riddler in '*Batman*'.

'*The Graduate*', with Dustin Hofmann as a young man who refuses to surrender to the older generation's rules, is another example of a film with the Argon theme of a youth's conflict with adulthood (see Meditation proving in Chapter 9).

The Walt Disney Company has produced several Argon related movies. '*The Little Mermaid*', based on a story by Hans Christian Andersen, features a young mermaid, who is willing to give up her life in the sea and her identity as a mermaid to gain the love of a human prince. The themes of an amphibious mermaid and her transformation from sea to land creature are prominent aspects of Argon, as is the happy marriage (at a very young age) to the prince. Most Disney films depict 'The Magic Kingdom' of youth and puppy love.

Closely associated with both Disney and Peter Pan was Michael Jackson, the 'King of Pop'. His life story includes a constant search for youth through such means as plastic surgery and, allegedly, sleeping with an oxygen mask in an attempt to beat the ageing process. He named his fantasy-land home, containing amusement park rides and a zoo, 'Neverland'. Like many of our Argon characters, he died prematurely: the only real way to beat time.

The Eye of Argon

'The worst novel ever written', is the quip that earned *The Eye of Argon* its fame. The book has been subject to academic research and much jovial discussion on the internet. A favourite party game is to take turns reading the novel aloud until the reader bursts out laughing, at which point he or she loses. This criticism is not exactly fair, as the author, Jim Theis, was sixteen at the time he wrote the '*Eye*'. He died young, but retained the notoriety of being the worst author ever. This mocking attitude is propagated by a group of pompous adult intellectuals making fun of a kid who dared to try. Nevertheless, it is an entertaining read that depicts the Argon image of a naive fun-loving hero, capable, youthful and independent, a killer of enemies and conqueror of women. This romantic hero is a theme in both the Argon proving and Argon cases – a young, strong, handsome, capable, clever, fighting male hero (see Chapter 13, Case 1). The following passage from '*The Eye of Argon*', below demonstrates both the Argon hero archetype and the naïve writing style typical of the Argon teenager. Reading the rest of the book highlights many other Argon themes.

Presented with original typos – enjoy!

THE EYE OF ARGON

by Jim Theis

The weather beaten trail wound ahead into the dust racked climes of the barren land which dominates large portions of the Norgolian empire. Age worn hoof prints smothered by the sifting sands of time shone dully against the dust splattered crust of earth. The tireless sun cast its parching rays of incandescense from overhead, half way through its daily revolution. Small rodents scampered about, occupying themselves in the daily accomplishments of their dismal lives. Dust sprayed over three heaving mounts in blinding clouds, while they bore the burdonsome cargoes of their struggling overseers.

"Prepare to embrace your creators in the stygian haunts of hell, barbarian", gasped the first soldier.

"Only after you have kissed the fleeting stead of death, wretch!" returned Grignr.

A sweeping blade of flashing steel riveted from the massive barbarians hide enamelled shield as his rippling right arm thrust forth, sending a steel shod blade to the hilt into the soldiers vital organs. The disembowelled mercenary crumpled from his saddle and sank to the clouded sward, sprinkling the parched dust with crimson droplets of escaping life fluid.

The enthused barbarian swivelled about, his shock of fiery red hair tossing robustly in the humid air currents as he faced the attack of the defeated soldier's fellow in arms.

"Damn you, barbarian" Shrieked the soldier as he observed his comrade in death.

A gleaming scimitar smote a heavy blow against the renegade's spiked helmet, bringing a heavy cloud over the Ecordian's misting brain. Shaking off the effects of the pounding blow to his head, Grignr brought down his scarlet streaked edge against the soldier's crudely forged hauberk, clanging harmlessly to the left side of his opponent. The soldier's stead whinnied as he directed the horse back from the driving blade of the barbarian. Grignr leashed his mount forward as the hoarsely piercing battle cry of his wilderness bred race resounded from his grinding lungs.

A twirling blade bounced harmlessly from the mighty thief's buckler as his rolling right arm cleft upward, sending a foot of blinding steel ripping through the Simarian's exposed gullet. A gasping gurgle from the soldier's writhing mouth as he tumbled to the golden sand at his feet, and wormed agonizingly in his death bed.

Grignr's emerald green orbs glared lustfully at the wallowing soldier struggling before his chestnut swirled mount. His scowling voice reverberated over the dying form in a tone of mocking mirth. "You city bred dogs should learn not to antagonize your better." Reining his weary mount ahead, Grignr resumed his journey to the Noregolian city of Gorzam, hoping to discover wine, women, and adventure to boil the wild blood coursing through his savage veins.

Flatland

In 1884 Edwin Abbott, an English schoolmaster, wrote *Flatland: A Romance of Many Dimensions*.[i] Abbott used the exploration of dimensions to critique the social hierarchy of Victorian culture.

Flatland is a two-dimensional world where the characters are geometrical shapes. The narrator, a teacher, is a simple 'Square'. When the Square first meets a three-dimensional being, the Sphere, he finds it impossible to comprehend this phenomenon.

> It was the last day of the 1999th year of our era. The pattering of the rain had long ago announced nightfall; and I was sitting in the company of my wife,

---

[i] For more information see Sherr J. *The Noble Gases: Neon*. Glasgow: Saltire Books, 2016. A free copy of *Flatland* is available online at: https://tinyurl.com/68km5t

musing on the events of the past and the prospects of the coming year, the coming century, the coming Millennium. . . .

. . . Straightway I became conscious of a Presence in the room, and a chilling breath thrilled through my very being . . .

Sphere. Tell me, Mr. Mathematician; if a Point moves Northward, and leaves a luminous wake, what name would you give to the wake?

I. A straight Line.

Sphere. And a straight Line has how many extremities?

I. Two.

Sphere. Now conceive the Northward straight Line moving parallel to itself, East and West, so that every point in it leaves behind it the wake of a straight Line. What name will you give to the Figure thereby formed? We will suppose that it moves through a distance equal to the original straight Line. – What name, I say?

I. A Square.

Sphere. And how many sides has a Square? How many angles?

I. Four sides and four angles.

Sphere. Now stretch your imagination a little, and conceive a Square in Flatland, moving parallel to itself upward.

I. What? Northward? . . .

. . . I groaned with horror, doubting whether I was not out of my senses; but the Stranger continued: 'Surely you must now see that my explanation, and no other, suits the phenomena. What you call Solid things are really superficial; what you call Space is really nothing but a great Plane. I am in Space, and look down upon the insides of the things of which you only see the outsides. You could leave this Plane yourself, if you could but summon up the necessary volition. A slight upward or downward motion would enable you to see all that I can see. . . .'

. . . An unspeakable horror seized me. There was a darkness; then a dizzy, sickening sensation of sight that was not like seeing; I saw a Line that was no Line; Space that was not Space: I was myself, and not myself. When I could find voice, I shrieked aloud in agony, 'Either this is madness or it is Hell.' 'It is neither,' calmly replied the voice of the Sphere, 'it is Knowledge; it is Three Dimensions: open your eye once again and try to look steadily.'

I glanced at the half-hour glass. The last sands had fallen. The third Millennium had begun.[6]

Song

This idyllic song can be identified with Argon. Hum it while you read.

What a wonderful world[7]

I see trees of green, red roses too
I see them bloom, for me and you
And I think to myself, what a wonderful world.

I see skies of blue, and clouds of white
The bright blessed day, dark sacred night
And I think to myself, what a wonderful world.

The colours of the rainbow, so pretty in the sky
Are also on the faces, of people going by
I see friends shaking hands, sayin', "How do you do?"
They're really sayin', "I love you".

I hear babies cryin', I watch them grow
They'll learn much more, than I'll ever know
And I think to myself what a wonderful world.
Yes, I think to myself what a wonderful world, Oh yeah.

References

1   Politz JC. Review: Movement of mRNA from Transcription Site to Nuclear Pores Available online at: http://en.wikipedia.org/wiki/Cell_nucleus#Nuclear_envelope_and_pores
2   Hockney M. *The Mathematical Universe*. E-Book. 2014. Available online at: https://books.google.com
3   The Tetractys – *Mathematical and Mystical Meaning*. Available online at: http://www.ka-gold-jewelry.com/p-articles/tetractis.php
4   Dismore J. *The 7 Steps in Alchemical Transformation*. Available online at: http://ordosacerdotalvstempli.net/seven.html
5   Best coming of age movies according to Dustin Rowles. Available online at: https://www.google.co.il/search?q=Indeed,+the+best+coming-of age+movies +are+almost+always+ fish-out-of-water+films%3B+the+water+is+our+youth, + and+coming+of+age+is+how+we+acclimate+ourselves+to+&ie=utf-8&oe=utf-8&channel=fs&gws_rd=cr,ssl&ei=EsuLVqDNM4P6Upvmh-gP
6   Abbott E. *Flatland: A Romance of Many Dimensions* London: Seeley and Company, 1884. Available online at: http://www.geom.uiuc.edu/~banchoff/Flatland/
7   Louis Armstrong lyrics. Amazon Music. Available online at: http://www.azlyrics.com/lyrics/louisarmstrong/whatawonderfulworld.html

16

RELATED REMEDIES

Nobles

There is a connection between all the nobles, and they follow each other well in prescribing. One could say that there is a gateway giving a direct connection from noble to noble. The 'Window of the Sky' in Neon gives a direct opening into Helium. In Chapter 17 'Trees of Knowledge and Life' we will see how they are gateways between Argon and Krypton. Krypton itself has many mentions of stargates.[i]

There are times, both in clinical practice and in life's evolution, that we can move directly between these remedies in a vertical line, rather than the tedious journey through the horizontal rows of the periodic table.

The following symptoms of Argon illustrate some of the similar themes that link to the other nobles.

When on the phone, a friend said my voice sounded like I'd been taking **Helium**.

Feeling as if I'm inside a chrysalis during meditation and about to burst forth. A beautiful feeling. (Neon)

Delusion I hear the phone ringing. Bells ringing. (Neon)

Feeling very sensuous looking at a clear sky, the stars, and an almost full moon. Stayed awake an hour, soaking in the beauty. (Neon)

Lying in bed looking at the stars. The plough is clear tonight and my mood feels very good. (Neon)

I felt I was deflecting work. (Krypton)

In mind's eye, I was witnessing the birth of the Milky Way pour across the skies. I had a sensation of recognition and respect in my inner vision, a huge door opened inwards to the left. (Neon, Krypton)

The Milky Way is the white road, the road of awe. When the Milky Way is lying flat, skimming the horizon, the area overhead is completely dark.

---

[i] From the 1994 sci-fi adventure film *Stargate* (MGM) and SG-1 television series, a stargate is a bridge portal that allows instant travel between distant locations.

This is the portal into which beings of other worlds emerge out of. (Neon, Krypton)

In tune with the infinite. The right angle in meditation. The angling is also about timing. Connected in a mutually supportive way. I am the Way, the Truth and the Light. Only time stalks them. (Krypton)

Delusion that, instead of hearing somebody in front of me, I heard from behind. (Krypton)

Delusion that, as I walk closer to the hills, they appear further away. (Krypton)

There were fireballs and meteorites, but you're safe in water. (Krypton)

Asked myself the question, is everything happening all the time endlessly and we only perceive 1%. (Krypton)

Honey

Honey has been recently proved by Camilla Sherr and her Finland Dynamis School.

Like Argon, honey arrests time. Honey is a substance that can be preserved for thousands of years. Provers looked much younger, felt more age-appropriate and more in the 'now'. Many slept a more deep and refreshed sleep, with less guilt about sleeping at any time at all.

Of course, honey is born from the third day, the time of flowers and pollination.

Gems

The Argon proving mentions several gem stones; jade, obsidian and rose quartz. In *Neon*, we learned about Jade's relationship to the nobles, as a gem that receives universal power through its alignment with the vertical axis of life that connects heaven and earth.

Jade came into my mind and I later found a piece, which I carried about during the proving.

Dreamed about jade and obsidian and their balancing qualities. I realised that jade is for the abdominal chakra and obsidian is for the sacral chakra.

I dreamt I was in college and an old male teacher was trying to help me with a problem I was having with scour in calves. He was wondering if I had tried all the acute remedies and I said I had. He then went off and brought me back two plants. One was an evergreen jade tree and the other one he called Gospel or Bible plant, I think it was.

Felt very drawn to using and holding a rose quartz stone during entire proving.

Germanium

Clinical practice has shown that Argon and Germanium seem to lead into each other and follow each other well. When the teenage Argon is forced into a frustrated adulthood, the sense of failure, guilt and suppressed emotions accumulate, resulting in a Germanium state. Argon's need to preserve leads to Germanium's tendency to suppress.

Polaris

Polaris, the North Star, is a timeless remedy. Situated in the noble axis of heaven and earth, all the stars revolve around it and mark the cycles of time, while Polaris remains stationary in its static centre. Hence, one aspect of this remedy is a sense of timelessness.

I don't want to know what the time is, I don't mind what happens minute to minute and I feel at peace.

Same feeling of absolutely timelessness, it can't be yesterday we came here; it seems impossible and today doesn't seem like today, it seems like long time.

A real sense of timelessness, very still and happy to be here, yet not wanting to move and create a change in that.

Dream – time is an illusion and time is a construct we need to agree upon for it to have any meaning.

Other than the theme of timelessness, Polaris shares with Argon the theme of a narrow passage causing lack of flow, the third dimension. Polaris provers often experienced or dreamed of constricted passageways, for example.

In a car and it was hitting all the walls.

Dream about second car a Jaguar driving and bumping into walls but nothing bad happened.

Driving a little car and it was jumping like it wouldn't go into clutch and it was hitting into the sides all the time.

17

ARGON MMM THE TREES
OF KNOWLEDGE AND LIFE

As we have seen, both the third period of the periodic table and the third day of creation relate to plants and trees. Argon, the perfection of the third period, represents the perfect tree in the perfect garden. We might say that it describes the Garden of Eden, with two ultimate trees growing in its midst, the Tree of Knowledge and the Tree of Life. In Jewish numerology the number 18 signifies 'life'; hence we may suppose that Argon, element 18, has a special affinity to the Tree of Life.

The following are interpretations of the Trees of Life and Knowledge, both as physical forms and as abstract concepts. Although the two trees have been examined extensively in biblical literature, I hope this discussion will offer a new perspective.

A homoeopath may ask herself, 'Why should this interest me? I am here to learn materia medica and solve cases'. This may be true, but by learning to see the connections behind and beyond a text, we can learn to recognise the deeper meanings within cases and remedy provings, as Hahnemann puts it, 'to perceive'. Rather than comparing external symptoms, we may acquire the ability to match remedy to patient at the deepest core, that which lies hidden beyond the mere story. This core is called 'the Secret' in Cabbala, the meeting point of geometrical shapes, simple pattern of motions, poetry, myth and spirituality. But let us begin with the simple story.

The commonly known 'creation of man' story in the Bible goes something like this. Adam was the first man, living in the Garden of Eden. He was lonely, so God (a male God), put him to sleep, took one of his ribs out, and from that rib he created Eve. They lived happily in the garden, eating freely from the abundant fruit. There were two special trees in the Garden, the Tree of Knowledge and the Tree of Life. Adam and Eve were forbidden to eat from the Tree of Knowledge, a sin punishable by death. Eventually the snake tempts Eve with an apple from the Tree of Knowledge (so it must be an apple tree). She eats it, finds it tasty, tempts Adam, he eats too. Their eyes open, they realise they are naked and cover themselves with fig leaves. They also learn to tell 'good' from 'bad'. Bad Adam, bad Eve, very bad snake, bad sex. As punishment for their sin they are kicked out of the Garden forever. Since that time no one can find the magic Garden, but speculation is that it is in northern Iraq, one of the most war-torn regions in the world today.

This common version comes with many subtle variations. Most are as divorced from the original text as modern remedy essences are from their provings, resulting in the distorted modern materia medicas we have today. In both cases, Bible and material medica, we *must* read the original text precisely to discover the truth.

I will offer an alternative interpretation of this story, differing from the conventional viewpoint. Naturally there are hundreds of interpretations, but this one benefits from homoeopathic philosophy and provings. We will re-examine the biblical story from the perspective of this new information in order to understand this alternative version. First, we must consider that neither God nor Adam was male, and that the Tree of Life was initially invisible and non-operational. We must explore the ability of the trees to reverse reality, and perceive them as gateways between the third and fourth periods, i.e. the timeless Garden of Eden and the temporal and material world we now live in.

To understand the story more deeply, we will attempt to determine the species of the Tree of Life and the real meaning of its place *'in the midst of the Garden'*. We will look into the possibility that both trees, of Knowledge

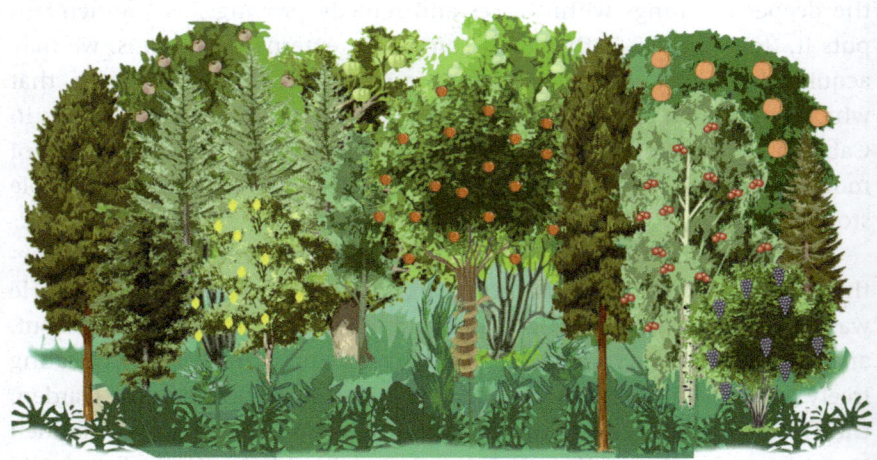

Figure 17.1 The Garden

and of Life, are one and the same, and that the Tree of Life is hidden within us all, ready to be found by those who seek it. We will discover the geo-metrical configurations and permutations that unite the two biblical stories of creation: the seven days of creation and the story of Adam and Eve. Finally, we will conclude that the Tree of Life embodies the Law of Similars in principle and function, and has bearing on our life at every moment. Thus, we are embarking on a search towards 'the secret', the place where all knowledge meets.

What's what?

There are two biblical creation myths that appear to differ in several ways. The first biblical story includes the seven days of creation and culminates in the conception of Adam. The second is the story of Adam and Eve in the Garden of Eden. Each features Adam, but as they are very dissimilar we must ask ourselves if this is the same Adam?

Who's who?

The first Adam was not male. S/he was a man and woman conjoined in one being. Notice the plural language used in the following Biblical verse:

> ... **Male and female** created He them.

It seems that God too was plural, as s/he creates the hermaphroditic Adam in his/her image:

> And God said: 'Let **us** make man in **our** image, after **our** likeness;

Note that in Hebrew Adam does not mean 'male man' but rather 'human being' (the Hebrew word 'adama' is earth, and 'dam' is blood, hence Adam is derived from 'blood of earth'). The translation of 'let us make man' is misleading. It should say 'Let us make human'.

Seeing Adam as male is a simplistic and patriarchal notion. From a Biblical point of view Adam was a hermaphroditic being containing both woman and man. Woman was part of Adam from the beginning, and was extracted whole from within him-her, despite the English text claiming she was 'taken out of man'.

> This is now bone of my bones, and flesh of my flesh; she **shall be called Woman**, because she was taken out of Man.

This translation is erroneous. The original text clearly states that Woman was extracted from within A-dam or human and not from within 'Male'. After this extraction 'Adam' remained as a word for the now-emptied out man, while she got a new name: Wo-man. Woman was not called 'Eve' at this stage; it is only at the end of the story that she gets her name.

There was no 'male' Adam first, followed by rib, followed by Eve. This is a reduction into 'cause creates effect' rather than 'two interconnected phenomena', which is one of the banes of modern science.

We have learnt that God embodies both male and female principles, and that **He-She** created **A-dam** in **their** image. **God and First Human are whole and genderless.** Adam was hermaphroditic, containing both male and female within (Helium). Woman was extracted from within this whole human being. Now they are two halves, rather than one whole. We will later see how this works schematically.

What exactly was forbidden?

God plants the beautiful Garden of Eden, filled with every kind of tree, including the Trees of Life and Knowledge. Although both trees are present, strangely it is only the Tree of Knowledge that God forbids Adam to eat. God does not forbid Adam to eat from the Tree of Life. Inexplicably, it is never mentioned to the Adams.

> And the LORD God commanded the man, saying: 'Of every tree of the garden thou mayest freely eat; but of the tree of the knowledge of good and evil, thou shalt not eat of it; for in the day that thou eatest thereof thou shalt surely die.[1]

The punishment for eating the fruit of the Tree of Knowledge is death. It is common to think that Adam and Eve's punishment was to be banished from the Garden. The Biblical text shows differently. According to the text, they are banished as a precaution against eating from the Tree of Life and becoming God-like.

> For the man has **become one of us to know good from bad**, and now he will send forth his hand and **take from the tree of life and live forever**. Therefore the LORD God sent him forth from the Garden of Eden, to till the ground from whence he was taken.[2]

Adam, Eve and the snake *do* receive punishment for eating from the Tree of Knowledge: hard labour for Adam, hard labour for Eve, crawling the earth for the snake, but not banishment (and not death either!). Banishment is to prevent them from eating the Tree of Life fruits, becoming God-like and living forever.

The question arises – Why does God *not* forbid humans to eat from the Tree of Life, but later banishes them in case they will eat from this tree? There are two possible reasons.

The first possibility is that prior to eating from the Tree of Knowledge Adam and Woman are already immortal. According to the text they will die only after they eat of the Tree of Knowledge.

> But of the tree of the knowledge of good and evil, thou shalt not eat of it; for in the day that thou eatest thereof thou shalt surely die.

We can conclude that Adam and Woman will live forever anyway. After all they are created in God's image. There would therefore be nothing to gain from eating of the Tree of Life. If they are immortal, why should they bother? Even if they do eat from its fruit, nothing would change. No need for God to worry.

The second possible reason that God does not mention the Tree of Life or warn Adam and Woman to abstain from eating its fruit is that it is **not necessary**, because **they do not know the Tree of Life exists**. We know from the text that the Tree was present in the Garden, so how could Adam and Woman not know that it was there? The only possible reason is that **Tree of Life is invisible** to them until the moment they gain knowledge. Before knowledge their eyes are not yet open to see it. They are blinded by innocence, and do not see that which they do not have any concept of, just as the native Americans looked at the first European boats approaching their shores but did not see them. The notion of 'ship' was too foreign to the natives. Like an Argon child, Adam and Woman feel immortal, deaf to the ticking clock of death. Like a teenager, they believe they will live forever. There is no time, hence there is no death. Life is preserved in its fullness and perfection. They embody the Tree of Life, and precisely because of this, they cannot see it.

Though we, the readers, know from the beginning that the Tree of Life exists, the best way for God to protect Adam and Eve from eating its fruit is to make it invisible and not to mention it. Conceptually this is similar to saying they ate from the Tree of Life but nothing happened; they did not perceive its invisible hidden powers.

Why does God banish the Adams instead of simply forbidding them to eat from the Tree of Life, now that they can see it? Simplistically, we can say that S/he already learnt the stuff humans are made of – we crave the forbidden.

In conclusion, there are two trees, the Tree of Knowledge and the Tree of Life. At this stage only the Tree of Knowledge is forbidden. The Tree of Life is never forbidden, though God would prefer humans not to eat from it, or even need to eat from it. As long as Adam and Woman do not eat from the Tree of Knowledge, they are immortal. Before they gain knowledge, their eyes are not open to perceive the Tree of Life, and it would not work anyway, as there is no looming death. Even if they do eat from the Tree of Life, its powers are invisible to them, so there is no reason for God to mention or forbid its fruits. This is akin to a totally healthy person taking the ultimate remedy. Nothing happens. Only when they get sick will this amazing similimum remedy work.

Once Adam and Woman gain knowledge and realise the inevitability of death, they are then able to see the Tree of Life, and now God will have to stop them eating it. It appears that we humans may either have immortality or knowledge, but not both. We can only become immortal again by losing knowledge, and that is not an easy feat. Seeing we have gained knowledge, we should now learn its painful lesson. Adam and Eve are banished from the Garden, and an angel with a revolving sword guards the way back. The English translation calls this 'The sword that turns every way'. This is not precise. The original text says the sword that 'turns over', flips, rotates, reverses or changes. Hence the 'revolving' sword can be understood as a mirror. Whoever shall look at it will see himself only, and not the gateway to freedom that lies beyond.

Where are the trees planted?

The Biblical text states:

> ... the **tree of life in the midst of the garden**, and the tree of the knowledge of good and evil. . . .

God plants a garden, and *in the middle* of this garden is the Tree of Life. The Tree of Knowledge is not mentioned as being in the middle.

In this context *midst* means the central, vertical axis that joins heaven and mid-earth and with which we align in absolute health. This central vertical line is apparent in the all the noble gas provings. When we are aligned with it, we are filled with universal life, wisdom and strength. We light up, just as the noble gasses do when plugged into electricity. Before knowledge, Adam and Woman could not see the Tree of Life because it was within them – in their midst – they were in the midst, aligned and immortal. They could not realise they were immortal because they did not even know there is death. When we are in the 'Here and Now', how can we conceive of being in the 'There and Then'?

However, Woman meets snake and has a change of perception. Previously only the Tree of Life was said to be in the midst of the garden. Inexplicably, Woman now reports that the forbidden Tree of Knowledge is in the midst. It seems that the two trees switched places. Either that, or

Woman herself changed place. Somehow the serpent changed Woman's reality.

> But of the fruit of the **tree which is in the midst of the garden**, God hath said: Ye shall not eat of it, neither shall ye touch it, lest ye die.

With the Tree of Knowledge in our midst comes the realisation of death. Eternal life is no longer within us, it is outside, and the possibility of death has moved within.

Eternal life or infinite knowledge; these trees affect man so profoundly that they must be able to change our very DNA, the blueprint of our intellect, health, disease and lifespan. As an analogy, we may compare the tree in the midst of the garden to DNA, which lies in the centre of our cells, protected by a membrane. At first it is the DNA of eternal life, with no death programmed into its chromosomes, but then it changes, and like a serpent virus, the DNA of knowledge invades and overtakes the nucleus in the midst of our cell.

What are the consequences of this infection and how did the virus get in?

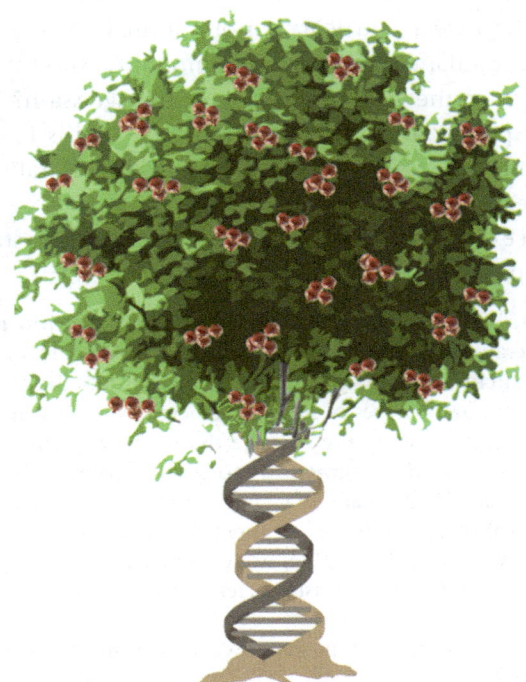

Figure 17.2 DNA Tree

After eating the forbidden fruit, why aren't the Adams dead?

Even though God promises that *'in the day that thou eatest there of thou shalt surely die'*, Adam and Woman **do not** die, at least not on the same day. Did God lie? Was Death an empty threat? Note that the phrase *'thou shalt surely die'* is an imprecise translation. The more precise translation is *'death you will die'*, OR *'dying you shall die'*, which means that 'death' will come into existence although physical death will not necessarily be on that specific day.[i] This meaning is confirmed later in the story.

According to most translations the snake reassures Woman that if she eats from the fruit 'You will surely not die'. This translation is also inexact. A more precise translation is: *'You will not die, deathing'*. The difference between 'die' and 'deathing' is like the difference between acute and chronic disease, quick execution or living in the shadow of death. After eating from the tree, there is certainly no quick execution.[ii] Rather, Adam and Woman now live under the vague threat that death will arrive someday – a much worse predicament. God's punishment has happened.

Let us look at this situation from another point of view. Was immortality really possible for Adam and Woman? Did they not have human bodies that are subject to wear and tear, poison, animals, viruses, weather and infection? What if Adam and Woman's immortality was not an eternal life, but instant death in the case of infection or transgression? You either live or die-but it happens now, in this very instant. Life is in the 'here' and death is in the 'now', rather than a prolonged deterioration of hopeless misery and disease.

Hahnemann expresses the difference between these two states as follows. Note words in bold:

> The diseases to which man is liable are either **rapid morbid processes** of the abnormally deranged vital force, which have a tendency to finish their course more or less **quickly, but always in a moderate time** – these are termed acute diseases; – or they are diseases of such a character that, with small, often imperceptible beginnings, dynamically derange the living organism, each in its own peculiar manner, and cause it **gradually** to deviate from the healthy condition, in such a way that the automatic life energy, called vital force, whose office is to preserve the health, only opposes to them at the commencement and during their progress **imperfect, unsuitable, useless** resistance, but is unable of itself to extinguish them, but must **helplessly suffer** (them to spread and) itself to be **ever**

---

[i] To better understand this concept read discussion at https://answersingenesis.org/death-before-sin/genesis-2-17-you-shall-surely-die/

[ii] The Jewish *Midrash* states that God postponed the punishment for a moment, a God moment, which lasts forever.

more and more abnormally deranged, until **at length** the organism is destroyed; these are termed **chronic diseases**. They are caused by infection with a chronic miasm.[3]

Here *death* is represented by acute disease while *deathing* is the lengthy and slow chronic deterioration through prolonged misery; the perfect moment of Argon versus the *slip-sliding away* of chronic Krypton.

And, according to Hahnemann, who caused all of this misery?

'They are caused by infection with a chronic miasm'.

Enter the snake.

The subtle snake

Here lies the tale of the animal that is all tail.

Now the serpent was more subtle than any beast of the field.

Subtle means crafty in a concealed way. The snake is going to convince Woman to eat from the Tree of Knowledge. What was so subtle about the snake's approach? Did the snake, as is commonly perceived, just lie to Woman that all would be OK if they ate from the tree? Such a crude lie would be fit for a hyena, kangaroo or even a human, but can hardly be considered worthy of the most subtle of beasts. In fact, it was not a lie because Woman and Adam did not die after all.

Subtle means telling a lie in a way that can hardly be detected, an expert con job, a magician gently misdirecting his audience. The snake's mode of operation fits precisely into the well-known stages of a sophisticated con job.[4] Let us examine his tactics.

Step one: Separate the parties. The snake knows that Adam and Woman together will present a stronger resistance, so he corners Woman on her own.

The snake also knows that the best lies are those closest to the truth, and that truth, if it is not the whole truth, is the most subtle of lies. For instance, is a snake all tail as written at the head of this chapter? Is that easy to believe for a moment? Wrong – a snake has a head. Nearly true, but not all true.

The snake in the Bible tells three near-truths. First 'the tease', meant to prime the 'mark' into a different perception and distort their reality. He (or she?) starts with an innocent general question.

Yea, hath God said: Ye shall not eat of any tree of the garden?

This is not true, but it focuses Woman on the forbidden. 'Did Mom tell you not to eat any of the food in house?' 'Errr no, come to think of it, she only forbade the chocolate. Mmmm ... the chocolate.' A simple change of perception. Previously the tree in the midst is the Tree of Life. Now the Tree of Knowledge moves to the midst of Woman's garden of consciousness, and she wants it!

> But of the fruit of the **tree which is in the midst of the garden**, God hath said: Ye shall not eat.

God forbade to eat of the Tree of Knowledge, but it was not in the midst of the Garden. Now it is. The forbidden 'chocolate' becomes centre of attention – the woman cannot stop thinking about it. The virus has entered the nucleus and it kindles a sense of lack that the snake can exploit.

Let us look at this subtle deception in another way. Maybe it is not the two trees that change places, but Woman herself. Initially she is in the midst of the garden, with a perspective of life, simply being, as central. Once she shifts her perception outwards she will think that the Tree of Knowledge is in the midst. Analysing, thinking and comparing will supersede being. We might say that the snake changed Woman's perspective to see herself from 'without in' instead of from 'within out (Figure 17.3). Knowledge takes primary position while being here and now becomes secondary. This false perspective is the result of Psora, a predicament we all share. We believe we live outside our eyes rather than within the midst of our being, and this breeds desire and envy. To understand this try to be aware where *you* live from – from the eyes outwards or from the centre inwards?

The snake now performs his second refined misdirection, known in con circles as the 'the please'. This means that the advertised deed is presented as legitimate and without consequence. The potential gains are exaggerated, risks minimized or neglected. Woman says: 'If we eat from the tree we will die'. To which the snake replies with the truth: '*You will not die, but deathing*'. Sounds close enough, and not too bad.

Will death occur instantly on eating the forbidden fruit? No, promises the snake. You have time. Mañana. It will be a postponed sentence,

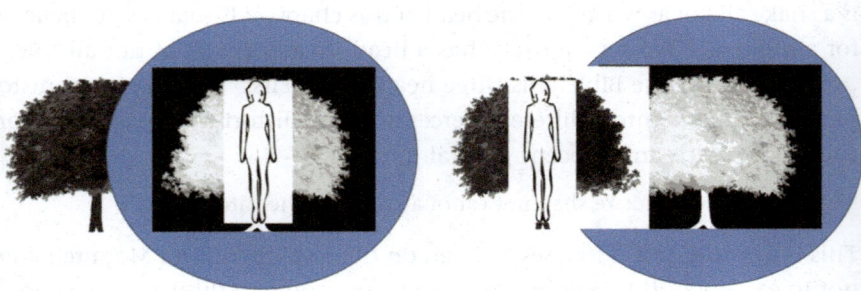

Figure 17.3 Woman in midst and in the periphery of the garden

prolonged but not immediate. This is the truth, but it is a dreadful truth. What the snake does not mention is that instant death would be far preferable to the Damocles sword we will endure in a chronically diseased life. But all Woman can hear is *'You will not die'*. This trick is the essence of addiction and allopathy. Joy and satisfaction now, pay the price later, much later. No worries.

Now for the third stage, 'the squeeze', where the 'mark' is promised a special and one-time only upgrade or bonus. The 'special deal' is that Woman and Adam will be like gods. The snake does not lie when saying they will be like gods if they eat the fruits of the Tree of Knowledge. Just as he promises, their eyes *will* open and they *will* know good from bad, and thus they *can* be like gods. This is entirely possible, as the text later confirms, God himself is aware of this possibility. The snake simply 'forgets' to mention that humans are not permitted to have both knowledge and eternal life at the same time and cannot become the one God.

Before eating from the Tree of Knowledge, Adam and Woman are immortal, but they cannot have knowledge. After eating, they gain knowledge but cannot have eternal life. Our fate is to choose one or the other, but not both. Immortality precludes knowledge, and knowledge harbours death. If we could have both together, we would be Gods, knowing all and living forever.

Woman was not convinced by lies. She was convinced by near truths and partial truths, tales without a head. This is a susceptibility we suffer from to this very day. Seven billion people on this planet are being conned every day, every moment in this very way. Just ask Big Pharma how they

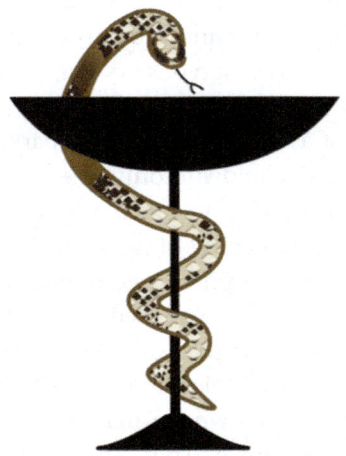

Figure 17.4 Big Pharma logo

convince people to take their venomous vaccinations and appalling drugs. It is true that many times these venoms save us from immediate death, but the dreadful unmentioned price is 'deathing'. Drugs protect us from death, but condemn us to deep chronic suffering. We have been saved from small pox, but now we have a planet rife with autism, cancer, diabetes, depression and dementia.

Like the snake, Big Pharma promises pleasure today and 'side effects' tomorrow, saving your life in exchange for long-term disease. And today, in the early 21th century, it promises us that if we only let it into our DNA, we can be like gods.

Enter the snake. No wonder he is condemned to live in the dirt.

How does the fruit work?

How did a simple fruit cause such a profound change? Do not be fooled by the notion that Adam and Woman had to eat from the fruit; it appears that touching it will do the trick. Woman declares that:

> God hath said: Ye shall not eat of it, **neither shall ye touch it**, lest ye die.

It is not clear from the text if God forbade Adam and Woman to touch the fruit or if it is Woman's interpretation, but it seems more likely to be God's decree. Why would Woman invent such an edict. If the fruit does impart its knowledge via touch we can conclude that it operates through the nervous system rather than the digestive system. This is a matter of contacting a vital current, not swallowing some kind of 'knowledge vitamin' that slowly percolates through our digestive system into our blood. The instant change that occurs when Adam and Woman eat the fruit confirms that it does indeed work through the nervous system.

A mere touch is enough to trigger the electrical charge needed to spark the nervous system, just as static electricity is sparked after touching wool. Hahnemann states that the midwife only need touch the baby to give it Psora, and we know it is enough to touch a remedy to get a dose; there is no need to swallow it. The opening of Adam and Woman's eyes is instant, and as such is reminiscent of a potentised remedy's action.

The real action of the Tree of Knowledge is to reverse the direction of time-space flow from life-wards to death-wards. But the change is not in universal time-space direction. Nothing changes in the external world; rather it is a polarity flip in our own bio-magnetic-electric current, a change in the direction of our vital force's spin. This change puts us at odds with universal time flow.

To summarise, the infection with knowledge, stimulated by touching the fruit, causes a change of direction in the vital current. This immediate action is akin to that of a remedy. The Tree of Knowledge is potentised. Does this mean that it also has similar properties?

Which tree is the Tree of Knowledge?

According to various Christian traditions and art, the Tree of Knowledge is an apple tree. This is highly unlikely and probably based on a Latin pun, conflating apple and evil.[5] There are a number of other theories which include pomegranate, fig, carob, citron, pear and mushrooms. If we look to the foods known in biblical times as the seven species of food, wheat, barley, grape, fig, pomegranates and date, that leaves pomegranate and fig to consider.[i] The carob and pear are never mentioned in the Bible. I will later argue that the fig is the Tree of Life, and so we will examine the pomegranate as the Tree of Knowledge.

A symbol of fertility, the pomegranate is native to modern-day Iran and Iraq, the region of the Garden of Eden. The proving of Pomegranate is full of sensuality, temptation, ego, hormones and references to the painful departure from heaven.[ii] Note that the word 'pomme' means apple.

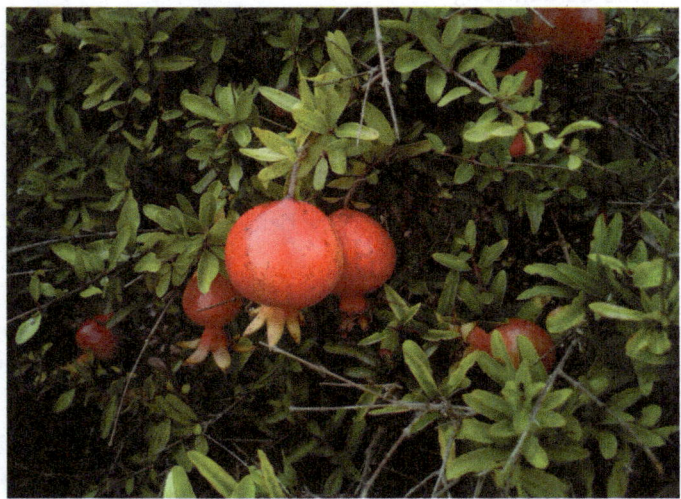

Figure 17.5 Pomegranate fruits. Tempting!

---

[i] Although personally I do like the view of American ethnobotanist Terence Mckenna that it was psilocybin, the bearer of alien knowledge, we cannot consider that a Middle-East fruit.

[ii] From the unpublished proving of Pomegranate by Dynamis School in 2004.

From the proving of Pomegranate:

I kept getting this recurring thought: 'In the beginning God created the heaven and earth.' It kept playing like a record in my mind.

Feeling like I'm in two worlds, slipping easily from one to other, like living in the waves.

Lots of sadness, past dipping in and out, each era, past childhood, sadness, weight, of futility.

Started to feel a lot of sadness, cosmic sadness, foreboding, everything made me sad, deep sadness.

Powerful dream: Making love naked on floor, sensual, appreciating each other's bodies, people filed in, his ancestors stood around watching us appreciate each other, full of sensuality.

Many sexual, sensual dreams, desire wanting exchange, focused on the feeling of sensuality.

Finally, we find the following ode to pomegranate in the "Garden Song" from ancient Egyptian hieroglyphics.[7] The negative aspects of measuring and comparing ourselves to others are very obvious in the pomegranate's attitude.

The Garden Song

The pomegranate speaks:
My leaves are like your teeth
My fruit like your breasts.
I, the most beautiful of fruits,
Am present in all weathers, all seasons
As the lover stays forever with the beloved,
Drunk on 'shedeh' and wine.

All the trees lose their leaves, all
Trees but the pomegranate.
I alone in all the garden lose not my beauty,
I remain straight.
When my leaves fall,
New leaves are budding.

First among fruits
I demand that my position be acknowledged,
I will not take second place.
And if I receive such an insult again
You will never hear the end of it . . .

What is the result of eating the fruit of knowledge?

After eating the fruit of knowledge, Adam and Woman are banished from the garden into a world defined by sex, death and procreation. It is clear that these three factors did not exist before.

Adam and Woman now see that they are naked. Sexuality appears, and for the first time they feel shame and cover themselves. The fruit also brings the vague threat that death will arrive someday. The only way for Adam and Woman to defend themselves from this future death and consequent extinction is to procreate. But while sex is mostly fun and procreation occasionally fulfilling, they both carry a price. Eve will have to suffer the pains of childbirth and childrearing, Adam will have to get a mortgage and sustain a family. This was certainly not the case beforehand.

When you cannot live forever you need to breed to continue the species, else it will become extinct after one generation. Conversely, if you are going to live forever you better not procreate, as the planet will fill up pretty quickly and you might end up living in your great-great grandparents' tiny apartment with an extremely large family. Preservation or procreation: Preserve eternal life or multiply and die – that is the evolutionary choice, the Argon dilemma.

Here is another analogy to look at this dilemma. At some point in the evolution of life on Earth, a mutation brought about change from mitosis to meiosis. The first brings about immortality by cloning, i.e. 'I might have a new body but it's still the same old me', while the second breeds sexually, creating variety and death, in other words, 'Over my dead body will I be like my father!'

This development corresponds to Day Three of creation. On this day, the day of the tree, seeds are created, which means that life can procreate but must also die. Seeds arise from the death of the fruit that bears them. The proving of Argon has many references to seeds and death, along with the desperate attempt to preserve life. But Argon, the Eden story and Day Three also bring about a cure, for they expose the one tree that can reverse the deathly process of knowledge – The Tree of Life, now visible and available.

We will study the nature of this miraculous tree, but first we must examine the nature of this sexy but deadly knowledge.

What is this knowledge anyway?

Even before eating from the Tree of Knowledge Adam and Woman knew they were naked.

'And they were both naked, the man and his wife, and were not ashamed'.

Once they eat from the Tree of Knowledge their eyes open.

And the eyes of them both were opened, and they knew that they were naked; and they sewed fig-leaves together, and made themselves girdles.

If they previously knew they were naked, what asset did they gain once their eyes opened? The added ingredient is shame. What was this formidable power, the power to make them ashamed, the power that changed our world forever? What did they now see that previously they did not?

What they saw was that they were different.

One can only perceive differences by the *ability to compare*. She has breasts, he has a penis; he is black, she is white; you are tall, I am small; I am good, you are bad; I am rich, you are poor; she is smart, I am not. Enter shame, pride, low self-esteem, ambition, racism, attraction, jealousy, hate, war, time and death; and worst of all, perfectionism. All that is ugly in the world.

Even worse, they (we) learnt to compare 'good' with 'bad', resulting in morality. Morality breeds a lot of 'nice' things, but it also breeds condescension, guilt and war.

Therefore when Tao is lost, there is goodness.
When goodness is lost, there is kindness.
When kindness is lost, there is justice.
When justice is lost, there is ritual.
Now ritual is the husk of faith and loyalty, the beginning of confusion.
Knowledge of the future is only a flowery trapping of Tao.
It is the beginning of folly.[8]

The ability to compare is not however the primary force that comes into play; it has a mother. In order to compare we need to measure. What we gained from that forbidden bite was the *ability to measure*.

Before the fruit we could not measure, and so we could not compare. Now we can determine length, height, girth, weight, colour, intelligence, beauty, riches, disease, blood counts, the distance to the moon and more profoundly, time.

If we are in the 'here and now' we cannot measure or compare. In the 'here', we cannot measure length, width, height or bank accounts. We can calculate these only when we have stepped out of 'here'.

If we are within time, we cannot quantify it. We can only gauge time if we step out of it. If we could not measure time, we would not die. There is only one instance where time has no measure, and that is in 'now'.

As the saying may go, time is what happens when we split 'now', and space is what happens when we split 'heres'.

Eating from the Tree of Knowledge took us out of the *here*, out of the *now*, out of the *midst* of the garden: the central, vertical noble line zero, around which the universe revolves. **Living forever does not mean not dying, it means living 'now', and when the time comes, dying 'now'.** Measuring, on the other hand, informs us that time flies and that death is waiting just outside the door. This is the nature of prolonged chronic disease, forever living in the shadow and fear of death. It is this ever-present fear of death that is the hypochondriac mother of allopathy and the rich daddy of Big Pharma.

Ultimately however, knowledge, the ability to measure and compare, is born from division, from chopping unity into units, from stepping into diversity, '. . . *From the one to the ten thousand things*'.[9] Just before the snake appears, Adam takes the measure of the different beasts, giving each a separate name and with it a separate identity. Internally they are still united, but naming each animal is only a small bite away from world fragmentation. The susceptibility was there before the snake struck and before the fruit was eaten.

> The tree of life was
> Here
> Adam and Eve peeked
> At the tree
> At their naked selves
> Now
> Fragmented
> Into there and
> Then
> Knowledge arose
> So that
> Now
> They could
> Compare, measure
> Genitalia
> And bank accounts

Now that we, humanity, are fragmented, we cannot use the tools of division and measurement to find the way back to unity and eternal life. Compasses, maps or computers will not lead us there, though we persistently try. There is, however, a way to reverse direction towards Eden, towards an immeasurable world of no differences, no diversity, no comparison, no 'deathing'; a world of unity. This way is The Tree of Life.

What is the nature of this tree?

What is the relationship between the Tree of Knowledge and the Tree of Life?

The solution to the threat of 'deathing' that emerges after eating from the Tree of Knowledge is the other tree, the Tree of Life. This tree has the ability to reverse us back to the 'pre-knowledge', 'pre-death' state of eternal life, an opposite function to the Tree of Knowledge.

The Tree of Knowledge can be understood as a 'gateway' or 'Stargate' leading from the world of eternal life to a world limited by time and death, while the Tree of Life is a 'gateway' back to timeless life.

These two trees are inverted, mirror images of each other with opposite and complementary functions. One is a gateway towards division, knowledge, death and sex and the other a gateway to unity, innocence and eternal life.

We may think of the two trees as up and down elevators. In the world of eternal life the Tree of Knowledge is forbidden, to prevent us from riding the down elevator into a divided and constricted world. The Tree of Life is irrelevant- we can't go up when we are already there. Once we descend into a world of knowledge, time and death, the Tree of Life upward-moving elevator is applicable, but placed out of reach to prevent our passage back to immortality.

The Tree of Knowledge bestows us with logic, the ability to measure, compare, analyse, calculate, infer and deduce. As the Tree of Life has opposite functions, we may reason that it bestows us with non-logic. After all, immortality does not sit well with reason. Two other words for non-logic are paradox and magic. The flip side of logic is paradox, the gateway to truth and eternal life. Remember how it felt the first time someone told us the paradoxical Law of Similars, a magical, life-changing moment.

The Tree of Life is non-logical. To climb it we must choose paradox. Choose paradox and we will get magic.

What is the relationship of the two trees to the periodic table model?

Argon, relating to the third day, is the element of trees. Just as the two trees are gateways between the worlds, each noble gas represents a gateway to the period above or below it.

Via the Argon gateway we can descend into the fourth period. The fourth period represents the painful world of time and toil. Its remedies are often characterized by low self-esteem and social trauma. Step by step, element by element, this period reverses reality, changing the direction of universal flow. It culminates in Krypton, whose proving contains many images of time, knowledge, measurement, hard labour, mirrors, reversals, and crossovers, all accompanied with loss of love. Here are some tasters from the descent into Krypton:

No energy, sliding down. *"Slip sliding away, Slip sliding away"*

We as a couple have lost the love we had before the proving, and lost the love of God.

Time is not equal and there are still points for entering the Stargates. The concept of time has changed. It feels more as a continuum present rather than in compartments of before, past, later. I went through the ages of time. I wish I could go back in time. Losing sense of time, difficult to calculate time.

Do you know how they measure horses, in hands?

Disgruntled, irritable as soon as I walk into my office. I'm extremely irritated that I've got to do work that is not related to mine. Overwhelmed with things I have to do but can't get organized to do any of it. Lack of motivation. Embarking on another unnecessary task. Oh how can I be really free!

H and A are the same in mirror image.

PHAT! A word used to bring a corpse back to life. Also used backwards TAHP

The fourth period is a step through the mirror to a world where everything functions in reverse. Krypton is the final passage way out of the Garden to the lower world of chronic existence. It reverses the magical world of immortal childhood into the logical world of time and death. The angel with the mirror sword guards the way back.

But just as Argon is the gateway down, it is also the entrance back to the third period.

Argon contains, both the Tree of Life and of Knowledge, which are mirror images of each other. Argon's passageway between the third and

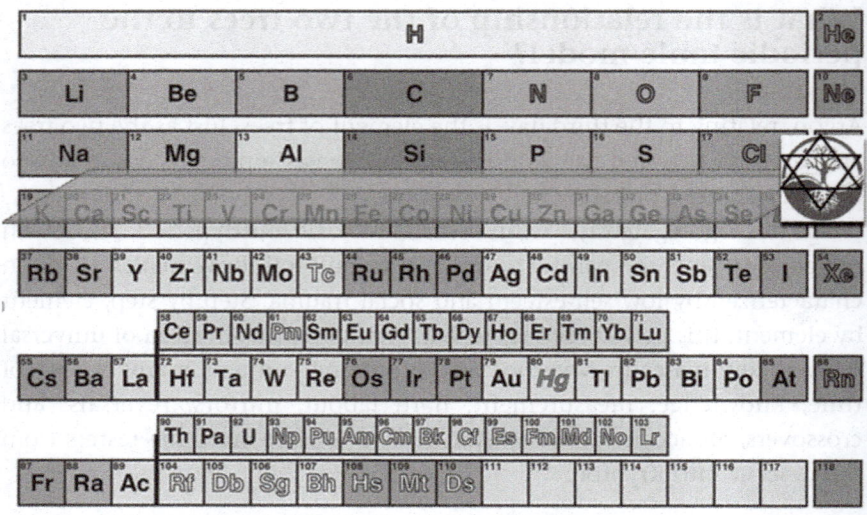

Figure 17.6 *A mirror separates the third and fourth periods. Argon is a gateway between them*

fourth periods transports us, via the Tree of Knowledge, to the lower world of the table, to the fourth dimension of time, work and death. But Argon is also the Tree of Life, providing access upwards to the third period, Peter Pan's world of 'timeless now'.

In Figure 17.7 we see Argon represented as The Star of David, a hexagon composed of two triangles, depicting the two gateways, one leading from up down and the other from down up.

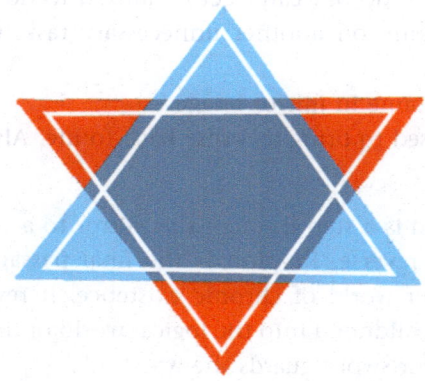

Figure 17.7 *Star of David – two gateways*

The proving of Helium gives us a glimpse at the magic we may experience when passing through the noble gateways, from upper to lower world and back.

I was in some Japanese-inspired surroundings. An egg-shaped pond with ice-cold water, and a thin layer of ice on top. I didn't know if it was muddy or full of plants, fishes, other creatures, or anything dangerous. I undressed completely and jumped in after a short hesitation. The others around thought it was a great, impressing, respectful thing to do. My body broke the ice as I jumped into the pool. The water was ice-cold but clear. I went all the way to the bottom, and was then rising slowly upwards. The sun was shining through the water making all the bubbles glitter. I had to take a deep breath while still under water, and found that I could breathe in the water. When I broke through the top it was like going through a membrane. I rose from the pond feeling like a new person, a cleaned person, actually more 'me' than ever. I was in contact with all of myself, and felt very whole. It felt like an initiation, and I was met with deep respect afterwards. Right next to the Japanese garden was a farm with a square swimming pool like an American swimming pool? People were swimming, screaming, shouting, laughing, acting rather hysterical, thinking they were having a great time. Some of them had been drinking. It all seemed very superficial compared to the quietness and spirituality right next door. But I felt I was a part of them too – or they a part of me. I knew what I wanted, and how I preferred to be, and which part of me I wanted to live. When undressing to go into the pond I felt very shy and naked; on rising from the pond the nakedness was spiritual in a way, with no shyness. (Helium)

What is the Tree of Life?

Finally, we come to understand that compared to the ordinary trees of this world, the Tree of Life is inverted.

Normally, trees function in an opposite and complementary way to humans. Plants breathe in the CO_2 that we exhale, and exhale the O_2 that we inhale. Their magnesium-based 'blood', chlorophyll, is very similar to our iron-based blood, yet chlorophyll is green and blood is red. Plants absorb our waste products, manure and urea, while we eat their fruits, which are essentially trees' waste products. Trees pump their food and drink upwards, while we pump ours downwards. Our lungs look like an inverted tree. Trees have their roots in the earth, while our roots are in heaven, from whence our soul descends. and in our brain, which is the root of our nervous system. This inverse relationship of humans to trees is confirmed by the following provings symptoms of Olive and Argon:

> Sensation of the soul leaving the body through the rectum. (Olive)
> Sensation of giving birth through the head. (Olive)
> When I woke, sometimes I would come into my body the wrong way around – either upside down, back to front or sideways on. (Argon)

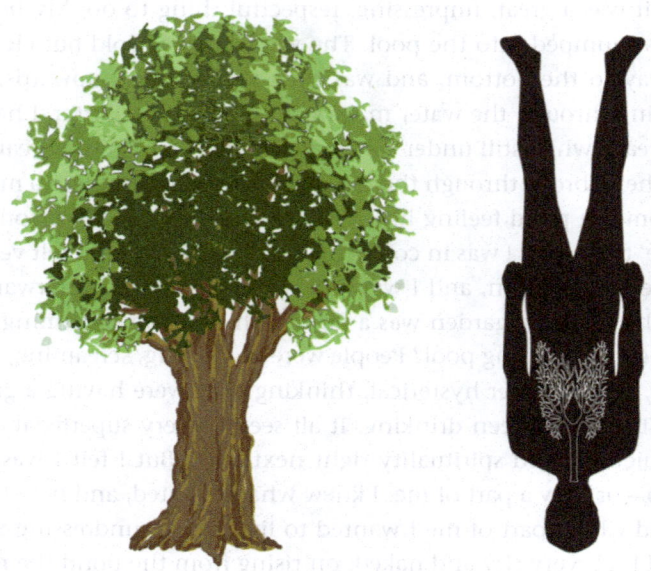

Figure 17.8 *Trees and human have inverse functions*

Thus, all trees have a reverse direction of flow compared to humanity. Except for one tree – The Tree of Life in the midst of the Garden. The Tree of Life is unique among all trees in its ability to do what no other tree can do – provide the passageway back to unity – hence it must function in a reverse direction to other trees. If all other trees flow in an opposite direction to humans, we can conclude that the Tree of Life flows in the **same** direction as humans. It is therefore the one and only tree that can restore us through the power of the similars, reversing the direction of our flow from death-wards to life-wards. This means that symbolically, or even in reality, the Tree of Life's seeds and roots are in the sky and its branches are burrowed in the earth.

There are a few species of trees that fit this description, but none more than the Ficus, collectively known as the fig tree, which often has aerial roots and earth-bound branches. It should come as no surprise that after eating the forbidden fruit, Adam and Eve cover themselves with fig leaves. As their eyes open the Tree of Life becomes visible, so they can use its leaves. The Tree of Life was, is, a fig tree.

Which of the many varieties of fig tree could it be? Research reveals two contenders: *Ficus religiosa*, the Bodhi tree and or *Ficus bengalensis*, the banyan tree. Let us compare them.

Ficus religiosa, also known as Bo tree, Peepal or Sacred, is the tree under which the Buddha sat when he became enlightened. It is said to be dripping serotonin, our natural, daytime 'magic mushroom' hormone that promotes feelings of happiness and wellbeing. A holy tree to both Hindus and Buddhists, it is the oldest tree depicted in Indian art and literature. It is said that this is the mythical 'World Tree' or the 'Tree of Life' of the Indian subcontinent and it certainly is a viable possibility for the biblical Tree of Life.

However, the banyan tree, *Ficus bengalensis*, which shares the features of its relative F. religiosa, has additional characteristics that convince us to choose it as the Garden's Tree of Life. First, there is an upside down structure to this tree which has an amazing canopy and size. Second, the ancient texts, Bhagavad Gita and the Cabbala contain discussions about this banyan tree in relation to the Tree of Life. Finally, the homoeopathic proving of Ficus indica, the common name of the Banyan, reveals links to the biblical tree.

The Banyan tree

Banyan or **Barh** *(Ficus bengalensis)*, belonging to the family *Moraceae*, is a remarkable tree native to India and tropical Africa. From the branches it sends down great numbers of shoots, which take root and become new

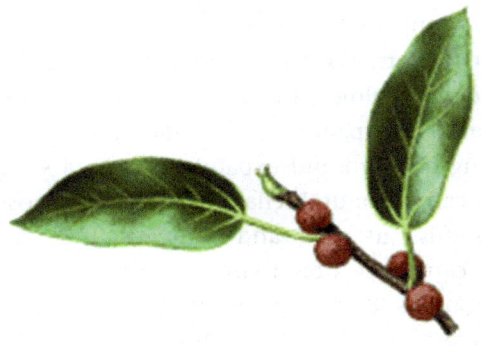

Figure 17.9 Banyan leaf

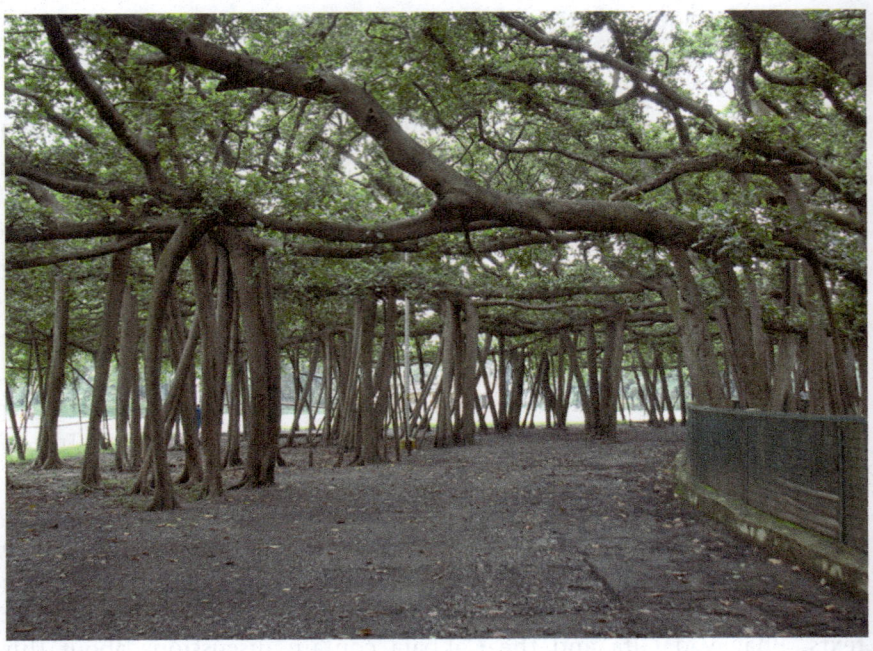

Figure 17.10 Great Banyan Tree

trunks. A single tree may thus spread over a large area and look like a small forest.

The world's largest Banyan tree, the **Great Banyan**, known as Thimmamma Marrimanu is located in India. Its branches spread over 5 acres, with a canopy of 19,107 square meters.[10]

The Banyan grows in a peculiar way. Birds drop their seeds into the top branches of other trees. The seeds sprout in the treetops and the banyan tree begins life as an epiphyte on the host tree, gathering its nourishment and water from the air as branches develop. Eventually, the lateral branches send roots down to the ground.

As it puts down roots, the trunk shoots up and branches spread out, stretching and bending, almost touching the ground. These reach into the soil, take root, pump up sap, and again shoot out branches. In this way the tree keeps growing outward and expands to form a small wood or forest under its massive canopy or umbrella. The host tree almost loses its identity as the Banyan sends out roots and branches. It is said that a mature Banyan's canopy can cover more than 1,000 feet in diameter.

The Banyan also has legendary and mythological significance in many cultures. This tree is sacred in many parts of India. In Hindu mythology, it is called *Kalpavriksha*, the tree that fulfils all your wishes. Hindu and

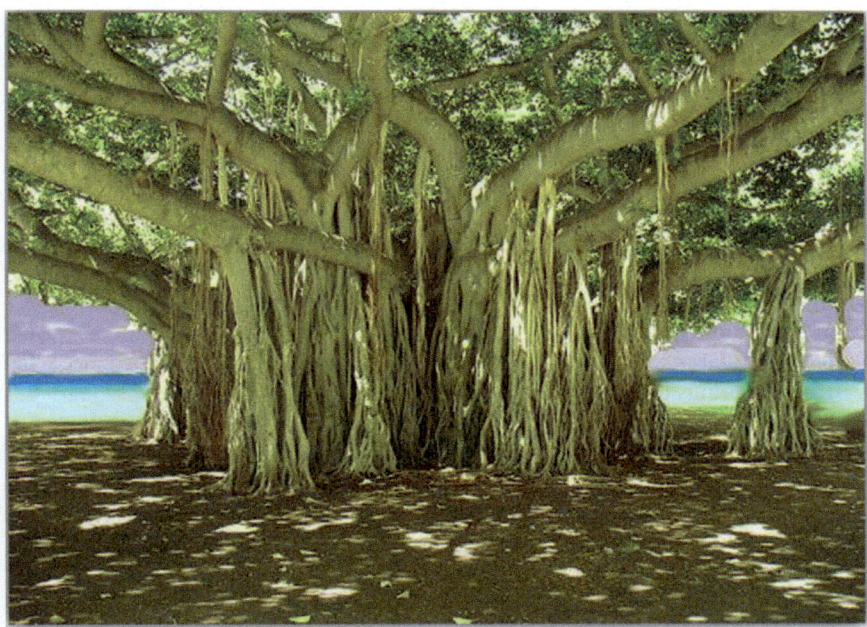

Figure 17.11 Banyan tree

Buddhist mythological tales and religious texts tell how Hindu sages and Buddhist monks sought the meaning of life and attained Nirvana under the Banyan tree.[11]

> Sages speak of the immutable ashvatha (banyan) tree, with its roots above and its branches below. On this tree grow the Vedas (scriptures); seeing their source, one knows their essence.
>
> The true form of this tree – its essence, beginning, and end – is not perceived on this earth. Cut down this strong-rooted tree with the sharp axe of detachment; then find the path which does not come back again. Seek That, the First Cause, from which the universe came long ago.
>
> Not deluded by pride, free from selfish attachment and selfish desire, beyond the duality of pleasure and pain, ever aware of the Self, the wise go forward to that eternal goal. Neither the sun nor the moon nor fire can add to that light. This is my supreme abode, and those who enter there do not return to separate existence. An eternal part of me enters into the world, assuming the powers of action and perception and a mind made of prakriti. When the divine Self enters and leaves a body, it takes these along as the wind carries a scent from place to place.
>
> Bhagavad Gita[12]

Rudolf Steiner explains this chapter:

> If we observe clearly we come to a place in the Gita . . . wherein Krishna reveals to Arjuna the nature of the Banyan/Ashvatha-tree, of the Fig-tree, by telling him that in this tree the roots grow upwards and the branches downwards; where Krishna further says that the single leaves of this tree are the leaves of the Veda book, which, put together, yield the Veda knowledge. . . . What does it signify, this pointing to the great tree of Life, whose roots have an upward direction, and the branches a downward direction, and whose leaves give the contents of the Veda? We must just transport ourselves back into the old knowledge, and try and understand how it worked. . . . The roots stretch far out into the distances of space and the branches extend downwards. . . . Remember what I have said in former lectures, that man is, in a sense, an inverted plant. . . . We then experience what this tree brings to light.[13]

In the Cabalistic *HaBahir* book, partly based on gnostic teachings, the Cosmic Tree of Life is termed 'KOL' meaning ALL. Its width and height are the distance a person can walk in 500 years and it is positioned upside down, with its root in heaven and branches in earth. Through its branches the heavenly emanations penetrate creation. The *Zohar* also describes the tree of life as upside down.

The proving of Ficus indica, the common name of Ficus bengalensis, was done by homoeopath Sujit Chatterjee.[14] In the proving symptoms we see the desire to care and nourish the whole of humanity. This extreme yin power of nourishment and replenishment is the essence of the Tree of Life, the very centre of humanity's common roots. Only such a power can provide everlasting life.

For grammar, brevity and clarity, the proving is edited into an *As If One Person* format:

I have deeper thoughts of life, health. I thought more deeply about death, especially the state of health and life. There is no use in being alive if you are not able to lead a normal life- you should be able to live with your total faculties.

I am at peace, nothing is really annoying me. Previously I was making a lot of fuss, nagging and fussing, but nowadays, I am at ease, because I don't think much.

Suddenly I realized that we are in the wrong place, walking towards in the wrong direction because we were talking about past and future.

A lady has a few months old baby and I like that baby very much and I always carry that baby everywhere I go. The motherly feeling is so strong I want to breastfeed that child. I hear someone say that it is not her child but she takes care of everyone's children in the same way. A very healthy feeling. It was not my child, it is beyond that. But the relatives say that she does this for everybody – everybody's children are the same for her. It is not just for this person or that person – It's the same for everybody's children. It's like she is viewing everybody in the same place, the whole humanity.

I see a big garden with many coconut trees, a very pleasant scene, and I was very happy to see that, a feeling of pleasure on seeing the garden. There is a big magnetic compass in the garden and beyond the garden is a sea and whole thing is very pleasant.

I have gone to a temple and praying in front of Swami Samartha and I am going in Samadhi and I don't know how long I am in Samadhi. I am not aware of the surrounding and I am in deep sleep and cannot remember anything, and when I came out of that state there is good calm feeling. Then I see my Guruji go and stand in front of the idol and I feel how come that person is standing there? It is a place for God.

My wife is admitted and some doctor is there and probably she has cancer. Her condition is incurable. I feel this medicine or chemotherapy, homoeopathy or doctors will not help her at all. Only one thing is going to help. I go to my wife and I say whatever name your Guruji has given you just take that name. That can do everything. Forget about cure of cancer. Your next birth will be smooth and you will go for the higher purpose of life. I feel as her husband, as a friend, as a human being, at the right moment, when it is needed, I have done the right thing. I just have full confidence in Guru and God; she was convinced with that and is going ahead with that.

A bus comes and knocks over a person and the man flies over from his scooter. I felt thank God, the bus didn't run over him.

A peaceful feeling like that of a child. No desires. Calm and cool feeling, great clearness of mind. No thoughts going in my mind. Improved concentration and lot of desire for meditation.

I have started giving to beggars, I feel their suffering. I feel I will take one dress less. But I will give to the poor.

No interest in work – Feel like leaving all this and going to a quiet place away from routine work, go to a calm and quiet place and lead a healthy life and be more independent.

A theme of trains has come up strongly – A train represents life. A train goes on 2 tracks, Similarly, life can be lead on 2 paths. One path is desire, ambitions, expectations, relations, friends everything. The other path is serving – you leave aside all this and are just serving. One has to decide what track he has to take. It is the point of realization; till now he has been following the track with a lot of desires, ambitions, and expectations and at that point he realizes it and feels like a fool for following this track. He realizes that we have been leading a life of expectations, bondage, conditions and he just leaves all that and crosses over and goes forward; much better serving. There was a pulling pain in my legs. I felt what you have to do when you leave these ambitions and desires and cross the track is to pull down your ego. Your ego should be pulled down to your legs. That is the place where your ego should be if you have to go forward and take up this path of serving the humanity as a whole – maximum strength.

This medicine has a lot of conflict between materialism and spirituality. I wanted to go further in spirituality and somewhere the other side was saying your parents have done so much for you and you have some duty towards them and you should do something for them, and that was taking me back from going absolutely spiritual. Spiritual means I will not think only of my family, not do only for them. The whole of mankind will be the same for me – any service to them. I will not distinguish that this is my father or this is my mother and do something more for them. I will do something for someone on the road also. I feel that my duty towards my roots is not complete.

There are people who are not aware of spirituality, the concept of life, what is life meant for? In this proving, everybody has realized – serving for humanity. This is the deep concept of life. Everybody has been talking at the level of soul. Not at the level of body. Awareness has come.

Dream my father is telling me to take "Hari Om" (God's name) constantly and I have a very happy, pleasant, peaceful, complete feeling.

Dream I am sleeping and covered with a blanket. People are coming and touching my feet and putting garlands on me, and I am surprised that when I am alive, why people are behaving as if I am dead.

Are there one or two trees?

From a literal viewpoint two trees are named and spoken about in the Bible. We even guessed at their identities as Pomegranate and Banyan. If we look at them from a larger viewpoint however, we can consider that the Trees of Knowledge and of Life are one and the same tree, but seen from different perspectives. When we are in Eden, near the source, we are on the path of eternal life. But from there we may see and are tempted by the Tree of Knowledge, offering the ability to divide, compare and desire. After traveling downwards on the path of knowledge towards 'deathing', we now see the Tree of Life and view it as our saving grace.

Perhaps it is just our worldly vision that sees these trees as Pomegranate and Banyan. We can never really see both trees as one tree in one time, but

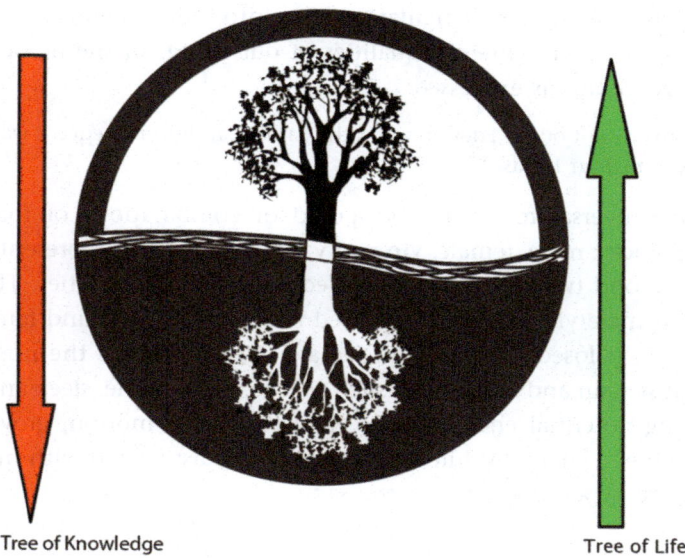

Tree of Knowledge   Tree of Life

Figure 17.12 *Tree of Knowledge inverse to Tree of Life*

from a higher perspective they *are* one tree, offering two inverse directions of flow. It seems that we can have knowledge, or we can choose timeless life, but not both simultaneously.

What are the evolutionary permutations from Tree of Knowledge to Tree of Life?

It is important to understand the following model as an analogy, a geometrical way to perceive the changes mentioned in the biblical story, but also a gateway to our search for meaning, life and health. While too complex for some readers, I believe this structure to be the blueprint of the Trees of Life and Knowledge, as well as the pattern that unites the two biblical stories of creation, the genetic sequence of incarnation, the process of meiosis and the configuration of DNA. Furthermore the model offers a key to the evolution of God's name in Cabbalistic terms.[i] If this is the case, then this sequence of permutations may have universal significance.

It is easier to understand this blueprint after reading about the sequence of permutations of the soul's evolution in *Helium*. Based on the Helium proving, it explains that as the individual soul separates from the cosmic

---

[i] Manuscript available by request from publisher.

sea of souls, the universal singularity splits into four individual soul parts, which represent the different qualities of our being. In the biblical story this differentiation is expressed:

> And a river went out of Eden to water the garden; and from thence it was parted, and became four heads.[15]

The four universal forces are composed of combinations of four basic building blocks: male, female, yin and yang. The first two represent gender and the second two represent concealed and exposed qualities. They can conjoin as male/yin male/yang (Closed male, open male) and female/yin female/yang (Closed female, open female). Yin represents the nourishing roots that sustain and rejuvenate, such as love, food, home, sleep and roots, embodying potential energy, while yang represents motion, growth and activity, kinetic energy. While the two forces are associated with male and female stereotypes, they are not the same.

Female/yin

Male/yin

Female/yang

Male/yang

Figure 17.13 Four types. Which one are you?

As the soul descends from the infinite to the material, the four qualities combine and recombine in different sequences, representing a variety of qualities and energies, which I have arranged in the permutation detailed below. In previous books of this series we compared this process to meiosis and the genetic recombination of DNA. This configuring of qualities also can be tracked within the two creation myths and the blueprint of the two trees. First we have a reminder of the steps of meiosis in these two diagrams, one simple and one more detailed.

We will now compare the formula to the blueprint of the two trees, to meiosis and mitosis and to the two biblical creation myths- the first of the six days of creation and the second of Adam and Eve in the Garden,

The sequence begins with the first stage of creation, Day One. The universe is invisible and dark, as both male and female **yin** forces are on the outside.

> 'Now the earth was unformed and void, and darkness was upon the face of the deep'.

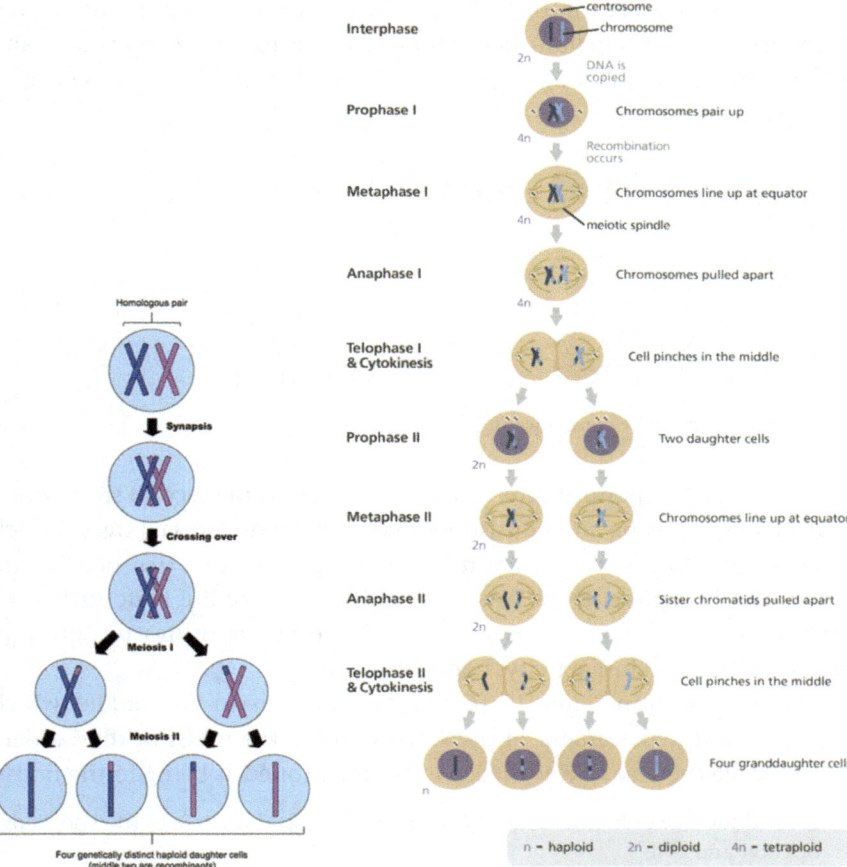

Figure 17.14 Stages of meiosis

All is concealed. It is a world of potential, a primary state occurring before creation; nothing has yet manifested. In the second story, that of Adam and Eve, the trees are not yet planted. Cells have not begun to divide (Interphase).

Female/yin   Male/yang   Female/yang   Male/yin

Figure 17.15 Yin forces on the outside

In the next stage of Day One, light is created. Singularities bang, hydrogen fuses into helium, stars shine. The yin forces move inwards and become hidden while the yang forces shine outwards. The universe begins to expand.

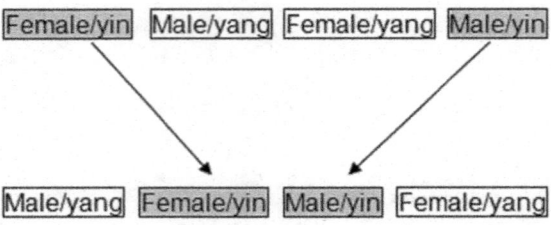

Figure 17.16 *Yin forces move inward*

This step corresponds to the Garden's creation in the second story, when God planted pleasing and nourishing trees and the two special trees. Which of these two forces, yin and yang, would represent the Tree of Life and which would represent the Tree of Knowledge? Since life is nourished by yin forces, the Tree of Life is yin. Knowledge brings things to light and generates motion and activity, hence it is yang.

As can be seen in Figure 17.16, the yin forces are in the middle, which correlates to the placement of the Tree of Life in the midst of the Garden. At this stage the Tree of Knowledge is not mentioned as being in the midst.

> ... and the tree of life in the **midst of the garden**, and the tree of the knowledge of good and evil.

This sentence corresponds perfectly to the sequence above. Being both hidden in the middle *and* yin, the Tree of Life is totally invisible, so that there is no reason to mention it or warn against eating its fruit. However, the yang and external Tree of Knowledge can be clearly seen.

Like the Tree of Life, the yin Woman is hidden and invisible in the midst of the hermaphroditic Adam. Woman has always been there, but at this stage cannot be seen, her name and identity entwined within the non-

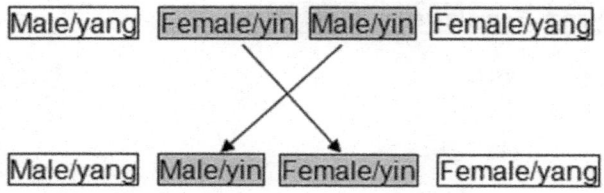

Figure 17.17 *Crossover of male and female*

gendered, a-sexual, Adam. Because the male and female aspects alternate male/female/male/female (Figure 17.16) there is no sexual polarity. (Prophase 1)

In the next phase of the Garden story, by crossing over the mid-sections, God extracts Woman from within Adam, resulting in two male forces on one side and two female forces on the other side; the first gender division.

This crossover is reminiscent of crossover in meiosis, the first mix. Crossing over moves sections of DNA between homologous chromosomes and allows for independent assortment and variety (Metaphase I, Anaphase I).

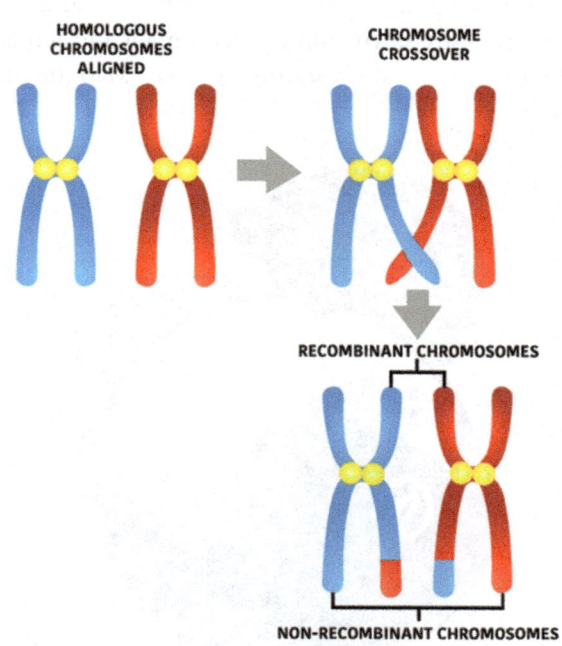

Figure 17.18 Meiosis crossover

In the next stage the Male Adam and Woman will be sawn apart, extracted from each other.

This is now bone of my bones, and flesh of my flesh; she shall be called Woman, because she was taken out of Man.

The Bible states the Woman was extracted from a rib of Adam, however the word for rib in Hebrew also means 'side'. According to Jewish lore, at this stage Adam and Woman were still joined together side to side by the ribs. God saws them apart and separates them, literally one from the other:

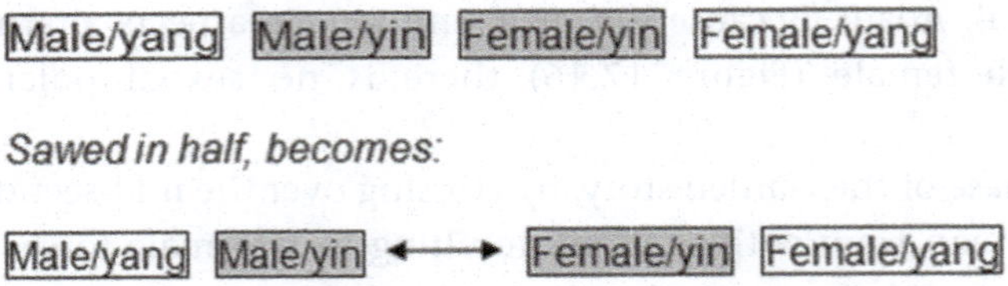

| Male/yang | Male/yin | Female/yin | Female/yang |

Sawed in half, becomes:

| Male/yang | Male/yin | ←——→ | Female/yin | Female/yang |

Figure 17.19 *Extraction of Male Adam and Woman*

a first step into separation and diversity. Note the similarity to the first meiotic division in Figure 17.19 above (Telophase I, Prophase II).

At this point in the Genesis story the snake appears, with its subtle power of sneaking into weak points and confounding truth and reality. It crawls its way into the recently-sawn split between male and female (Metaphase II). By cornering Woman and separating her from Man, he flips her perception of reality.

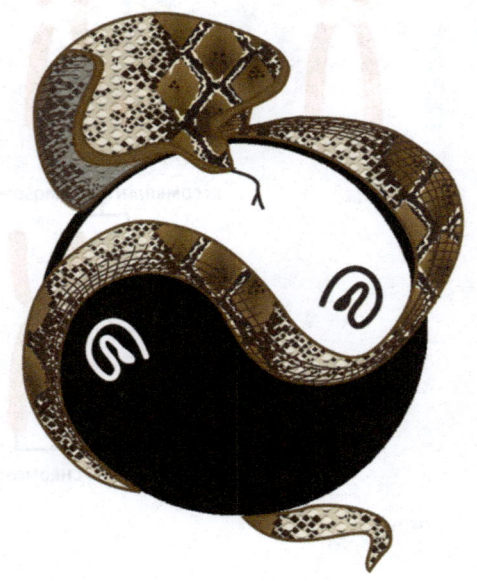

Figure 17.20 *Snake entering the spilt*

Woman's perception reverses and male and female yang move to the inside. Instead of the yin Tree of Life being in the midst as before, the adjacent male and female yang now bring the yang Tree of Knowledge to the middle. Because the Tree of Knowledge is yang, it is visible even though it is in the middle. Woman's eyes open and she 'sees' the tree.

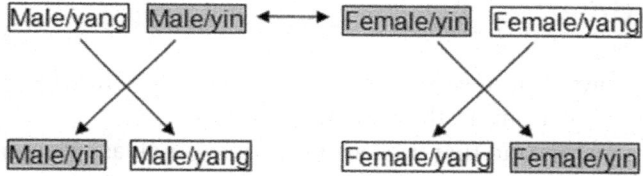

Figure 17.21 Male and Female crossovers

> And when the woman saw that the tree was good for food, and that it was a delight to the eyes, and that the tree was to be desired to make one wise, she took of the fruit thereof, and did eat.[16]

You have probably heard of the seafood diet – if you 'see' food, eat it. Woman and Adam 'notice' the Tree of Knowledge for the first time and do just that.

The resulting cross-over places the male and female yang aspects in the middle facing each other (Figure 17.21). Yang makes them visible and exposed and knowledge becomes the centre of their consciousness. Adam and Woman see each other naked and cover up. Knowledge is gained, but eternal life lost; sex is a bonus prize.

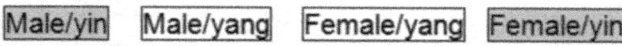

Figure 17.22 Yang forces on the inside

After separation Adam and Woman are two individual beings (Anaphase II). This final configuration (Figure 17.22) places the Tree of Knowledge in the midst of the garden, where it can be seen because it is yang. The Tree of Life is on the outside and hence can also be seen, but because it is yin, it is more difficult to find.[i] It is hidden behind the reversing sword, a mirror.

As we follow through a series of geometrical permutations, we see the four basic aspects of creation and of the soul (yin, yang, male, female) split, combine, flip and reverse, eventually shifting the Tree of Life, the 'here and now' of our existence, out of the midst of our being and replacing it with the 'there and then' of daily grind, the Tree of Knowledge.

---

[i] The final stages of meiosis (telophase II and cytokinesis), belong to Neon and relate to the Biblical story of Cain and Abel. Discussion can be found in the *Neon* book.

What is the time?

The Tree of Life's power is to reverse the 'deathing' process, which requires a reversal of time's flow from death-wards to life-wards.

It is essential to understand that the reversal of time is not, as commonly supposed, a reversal from future to past. The uni-directional arrow of time is a psoric delusion.[i] True time flows in a spiral or gyre. There is one *Now* that is in the centre with an infinite number of *Then* or *Future-Past* point possibilities in the periphery (Figure 17.23). To get a small idea of the infinite possibilities of future-past points just imagine the sum of all possible night-time dreams of everyone.

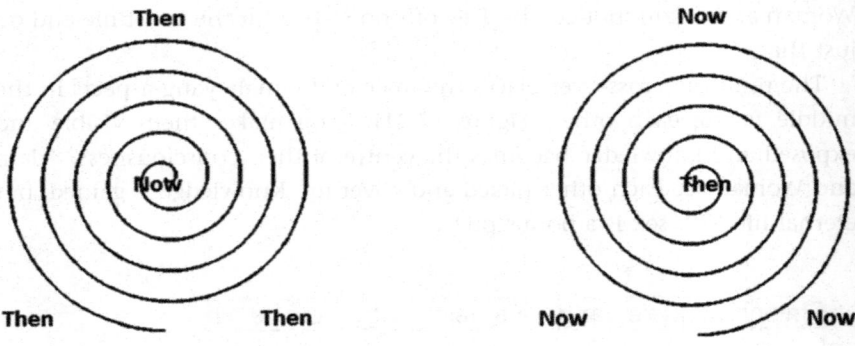

Figure 17.23 Time, now and then

This is in health; when we are centred in *Now* there is no 'deathing'. In disease, Psora, the configuration is different. *Then* replaces *Now* in the centre and time reverses the direction of its spiral flow (Figure 17.23). It is a small step out of our centre, but it changes everything. Our central position or identity is focused around *Then* or the *Future-Past*, while *Now* is banished to the periphery (Figure 17.23). It is due to this disposition that we are able to measure and compare – when we are *Now*-centred there is only one point of unity in our centre, so we have nothing to compare or measure against. When there are an infinite number of *Future-Past* points in our centre, there is plenty to compare. This is the true meaning of disposition. This change of consciousness can be caused by a mere touch of the Tree of Knowledge.

It is no wonder the first question God asks Adam after he eats the fruit is "Where are you?" Adam cannot really answer, because he is no longer in

---

[i] An extensive discussion on the subject can be in the next book in the Noble Gases series, *Krypton*.

the centre and has no reference point. All he can meekly say is that he is hiding because he is naked. He doesn't know where he is, but he can compare himself to his former state.

Once we become *Future-Past*-centred we are compelled to keep moving towards the '*There and then*'. The Tree of Knowledge is in our midst (Figure 17.24) occupying the central part of our being. From there it slices our perception of time into units that never stop moving. The clock ticks the seconds away and like hamsters on a wheel we run to catch up. The devastating effects of this can be seen all around us.

We mark and measure time; we live and die by it. We cling to the past and chase the future. We divide, we measure, we evaluate, we compare and we fight to prove which is best. We learn, we invent, we manufacture and

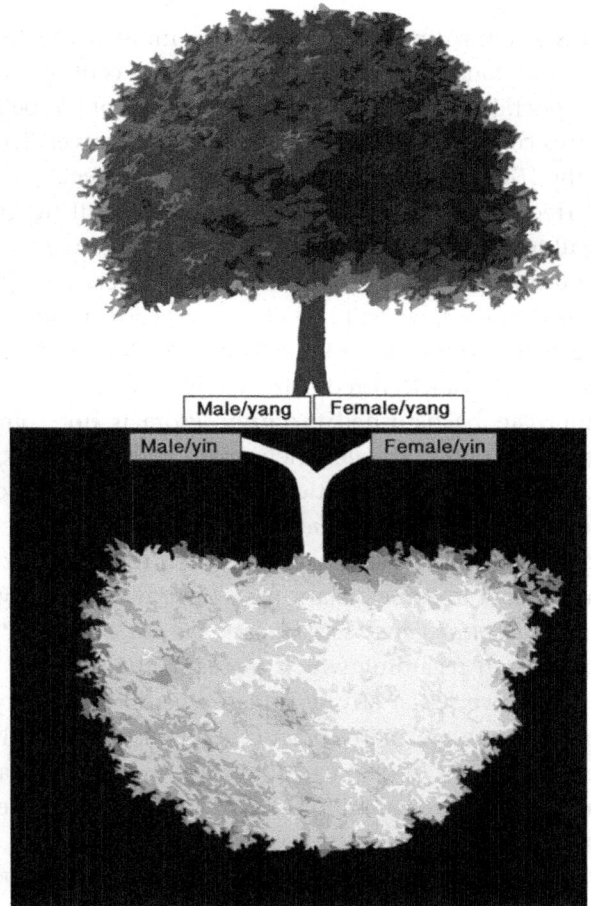

Figure 17.24 *Yang Tree of Knowledge in midst, Yin Tree of Life in periphery*

we consume. We feel empty, and from this emptiness a thousand diseases grow.

Action devours the hub of our lives. Yin, love, sleep, home and rest are relegated to the periphery as our life force is wasted on fruitless pursuits. We are 'deathing'. The Garden of Eden was the Garden of *Now*, but it has been banished to never-never land.

The Tree of Life is still there, but being yin, it is relegated to the fringes, where it is obscured from the majorities' vision (Figure 17.24). We will not find it in newspapers or on the television, in the stock market or in schools. It hides along the more difficult path, the road less-travelled. It belongs to the few, and is ridiculed by the many. It belongs to the fool with no knowledge. It belongs to the Joker, alone in a pack of hierarchical and competitive cards, but always adapting to the moment and eventually emerging the most powerful.

Our quest is to return the Tree of Life to our midst where *Now* resides in the interior of our consciousness. This is a dynamic central *Now* that flows towards a peripheral *Fu-Past*. With *Now* in the centre of our being, nourishing yin replaces consuming yang, and we may live forever. This is the real meaning of the *'Tree of Life was in the midst of the garden'*.

With the Tree of Life, the *Now*, in our midst we will never feel empty inside, but will forever be full and fulfilled. When we are once again nourished by the mother, when we learn to rest in her eternal time and flow from her central *position*, we will have lost our psoric disposition.

Just as the switch from life to knowledge is instantaneous, the change of consciousness to a *Now*-centred existence can happen in a second, and therefore Psora can be banished instantly. Psora is not something that happened to us 100,000 years ago when Adam and Eve were kicked out of the Garden. That victim-based notion is part of the psoric delusion, one that insists everything happened *then*. Our great grandparents did not get infected with psora, which they passed on down the generation to us. We did not acquire psora in some distant past. *Psora is something we create and re-new at every moment and every second, now.* We are 'Psoring'. 'Psoring' is a simple misperception regarding which tree is in the midst of our garden. As such it can be reversed at any second, a reversal of polarity – and it is easy to achieve. There are many practices, for instance meditation techniques and similar, that can help us attain this. The difficult part is staying there. The moment we are conscious of being in the centre, we are already looking at ourselves from the outside.

There is however one method by which we can reverse polarity on a more permanent basis, and that is by a similar polarity.

The Cure

Is the Tree of Life a possibility? Are we able to reverse time flow, restoring *Now* to the centre and *Future-Past* to the periphery? Certainly there are many ways with which we can turn around the consuming flow of time towards the rejuvenating *Now*. Two examples are sleep and meditation, both journeys to the timeless world.[17] They may not bestow full immortality but they do extend life and as such are a step in the right direction.

Every night we reverse time away from a fast-looming death. During sleep we experience 'healing time', without which we would live no longer than two weeks. Sleep can prolong life by many decades and is by far the most powerful life-extender we know. It is our nightly Tree of Life.[i] While today we live in the world and sleep a dream, perhaps in the Garden of Eden we lived a dream and slept in the world.

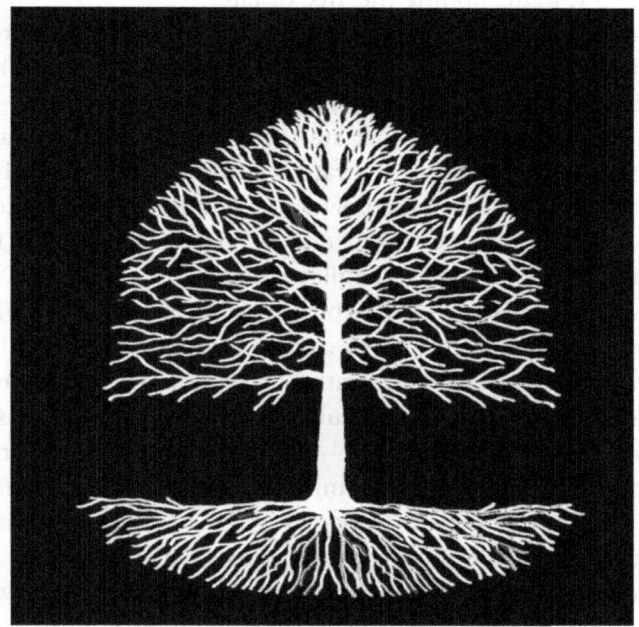

Figure 17.25 *Tree of Life*

What about the Tree itself? It is clear that the Tree of Life can change time's direction and restore *Now* to the centre. How does this magical tree achieve this alteration? The way to reverse flow is by means of a mirror. Light bounces off a mirror and changes direction, and therefore so will

---

[i] A full discussion on the nature of sleep appears in the fourth book of the Noble Gases series, *Krypton*, in which I attempt to prove that sleep reverses time.

space-time. Accordingly the Tree is some kind of a mirror. We have learnt that trees do not generally provide a mirror image because they are an opposite image to humankind. This makes them complementary but not similar. But the Tree of Life is unique. It *is* similar to humans, a mirror image reflecting the likeness of humanity and capable of reversing time's flow.

A mirror is not just a reflective surface. Mirrors, or similar reflections, can take many forms, such as words, sounds, images, poems, concepts or homoeopathic remedies. The *Law of Similars* is a kind of mirror, and so it is a method by which we can change the direction from death to life. The Law of Similars functions in the same way as The Tree of Life, rejuvenating and restoring our health by reversing time's flow towards the *Now* and bringing us closer to the present moment. This is the basis for 'Jeremy's Homoeopathic Law of Cure', *The true direction of cure is towards the here and now*. In other words, understanding and applying the Law of Similars is an essential step towards finding the Tree of Life.

The Tree of Life itself is hidden behind the gates of the Garden. These gates exist only in our minds; a delusion, smoke and mirrors. When we try to look through the delusion of these 'mirror gates', we see only our reflection, and ego abounds. To penetrate these gates, we must learn to look *through* the mirror. Hint: To penetrate a mirror you need another mirror. That which was reversed by the power of the snake must be re-reversed by the same power, by another snake, another mirror. To find the Tree, to go back to our source, we need to employ similars.

The reverse of flow is a change of perception in which the Tree of Life returns to our midst and becomes central to the way we live. It is a step back towards the primary configuration of the Garden, where yin is in the midst. This configuration may be found in sleep and dreams, in useless play, in meditation, in playing the fool – the power of non-doing, non-being; we may find it in the power of similars and high potency dilutions; the power of nothing. If we want to know where to start, try taking a long, useless afternoon nap in the middle of a busy work-day.

The Tree of Life is manifested in homoeopathy, not just by homoeopathic remedies, but in a homoeopathic way of living, of thinking, of being – a way by which yin nourishes from the centre, a way which returns us to the *Here and Now*. Because homoeopathy is yin and not seen by the majority, it may provide easy pickings for silly, yang bullies, but it will live longer and prevail.

What is the relationship between the Tree of Life and the Tree of Knowledge? Part 2

Previously, we said that the Tree of Knowledge was potentised, as its fruit can stimulate change instantly by a single touch, and we posed the question: Was it also similar?

From homoeopathic philosophy we know the following laws.[18]

1. A proving is a force (or remedy) that does something new.
2. A similimum is a force (or remedy) that does nothing new.
3. A proving is never a curing.

Because a proving is not similar to the person, it pushes us into new territory, i.e. into one of the infinite *future-pasts*. *As provers* we may become cats or dinosaurs or milk or plants. This may be pleasant or unpleasant, but because it is *new* we have a *learning experience* about the universe and ourselves. We do not learn from what we already know, we learn from what we do not know, and for that we have to step out of our comfort zone.[i]

A similimum matches us perfectly, and so there is no new experience, only a return of old experiences. Rather than learning, we forget. We forget we were prisoners of one of the *Future-pasts*, we stop running to the tune of *There-Then*, and we return to the *Here-Now*. The *Tao te Ching* states:

In the pursuit of learning, every day something is acquired.

In the pursuit of Tao, every day something is dropped.[19]

It is plain to see that the Tree of Knowledge is a proving, a dissimilar experience. It generates learning but not curing. The Tree of Life on the other hand is a similar. More than that, it is a similimum, and even more so, it is *The Similimum*, and moreover, it is *The Similimum for the whole of ailing humanity*.

But wait a minute. What is the Tree of Life similar to? It has to be similar to the effects of the Tree of Knowledge in order to cure or antidote its effects. It makes sense therefore that the Tree of Life is similar to the Tree of Knowledge. They are the same Tree, first creating knowledge and then antidoting itself. At one time we see the many branches of *Future-Past*, at the other the one root of *Now*.

We can only find a similar by comparing. We compare Pulsatilla to a person to see if they match. Are they thirstless? Are they weepy? Before we had knowledge, we could not measure and compare, and hence could not find a similar remedy, and neither did we have to! This is what is meant by

---

[i] 85% of all provers with whom I have worked said they had a learning experience.

the Tree of Life being invisible. Only after we do the proving of Knowledge and get the ability to measure and compare are we are able to find a remedy, in other words, to see the Tree of Life.

What is better for us humans – to prove or to cure? Curing is a wonderful non-experience, and forgetting our ills is bliss, but we do not learn and do not evolve in this way. On the other hand provings are misery, and although we learn, when applied continuously, they will wear us down. The process of evolution requires the correct balance between curing and provings. To potentise our beings God-wards, we need a good ratio between succussing ourselves with provings and diluting ourselves with Simili-mums. We need six days of work to one day of rest. We must proceed along each row of successive elements, as well as transcend through the Noble gateways.

This is why God decided to do the ultimate proving on us.

Thank God for the proving of knowledge, thank God for its cure. And three cheers to the snake (deep bow*).

We all know that the secret of enlightenment is to *know oneself*. In order for us to know ourselves we have to step out of ourselves, so we can measure and compare ourselves against the world. We then realize our differences. But when we have done that, we must step back into our midst again. And our midst is the same midst for everyone; it is our collective meeting point, the central yin in which we all connect and around which all revolves. When we look at the picture of the Banyan, we may think it is many trees, but it is really one tree. Like the great tree, we are one.

Both the Tree of Life and the Tree of Knowledge are available; we can choose one or the other, depending on how we view the world. We may evolve towards the fickle morality of good and bad, towards knowledge, science, analysis and division, and at the same time towards growth, learning and development. By using our logical minds we may reach for the stars. Or we may use the power of similars to synthesise and unite, amal-gamating our existence back towards one place and one moment. Like the androgynous Adam, containing both male and female, like two trees that are in fact one, the ultimate goal is to learn which tree belongs where and when. We must learn to travel both these paths each in the right time and ratio, harmonising one into diversity and diversity into the one. Then we will be God-like.

This is the secret of the tree.

References

1   Genesis 2:16–17 Available online at: http://biblehub.com/genesis/2–16.htm
2   Genesis 3:22–23 Available online at: http://biblehub.com/kjv/genesis/3–22.htm
3   Hahnemann S *The Organon of the Healing Art* (6th edn). New Delhi: B Jain Publishers Pvt Ltd, 2003 §72.
4   Chang KS. Four States of a Scam Available online at http://hubpages.com/money/Four-Stages-of-a-Scam-tease-please-seize-squeeze
5   Rupp R. The History of the 'Forbidden' Fruit. Available online at: http://theplate.nationalgeographic.com/2014/07/22/history-of-apples/
6   Deuteronomy 8:8 Available online at: http://biblehub.com/deuteronomy/8–8.htm
7   Pound E trans. *Love Poems of Ancient Egypt*. Hallmark Editions, 1971. This translation was based on Boris de de Rachewiltz' literal renderings into Italian from ancient Egyptian hieroglyphics on papyri and pottery dating back to 1567–1085 BCE.
8   Tzu L. *The Complete Tao te Ching*. Feng GF trans. Vintage Books, 1989. Available online at: http://www.wussu.com/laotzu/laotzu38.html
9   Tzu L. *The Complete Tao te Ching*. Feng GF trans. Vintage Books, 1989. Available online at: https://terebess.hu/english/tao/gia.html#Kap42
10 Great Banyan Tree. Available online at: http://www.atlasobscura.com/places/great-banyan-tree
11 Frank E. Multitrunk Trees and Other Forms. Available online at: http://www.haryana-online.com/Flora/barh.htm
12 Easwaran E trans *Bhagavad Gita*. Nilgiri Press 2007 Chapter 15.
13 Steiner R. The Tree of Life and Correspondence to the Human Nervous System in the Bhagavad Gita. Available online at http://aetherforce.com/the-tree-of-life-and-correspondence-to-the-human-nervous-system-in-the-bhagavad-gita-by-rudolf-steiner/
14 Chatterjee S. Homeopathic Proving of *Ficus Indica*. Reference Works Synergy Homeopathic, 2015.
15 Genesis 2:10. Available online at: https://biblia.com/bible/esv/Genesis%202.10%E2%80%9314
16 Genesis 3:6. Available onine at: https://biblia.com/bible/esv/Ge3.6
17 Lazar S. Meditation experience is associated with increased cortical thickness. *Neuroreport*, 2005 Nov 28; 16(17). Available online at: http://www.ncbi.nlm.nih.gov/pmc/articles/PMC1361002/
18 Sherr J. *The Dynamics and Methodology of Homoeopathic Provings*. (2nd ed) Malvern: Dynamis Books, 1994.
19 Tzu L. *The Complete Tao te Ching*. Feng GF trans. New York: Vintage Books, 1989. Available online at: http://www.wussu.com/laotzu/laotzu48.html

18

PERIOD III SYNTHESIS

We began our noble journey with the singular Helium individual soul, a one-dimensional perception represented by the crown chakra, the pineal gland and the 'third eye' (Figure 11.14). We then move to the second chakra and pituitary gland, where we split in two: backward into the subconscious shadows of our skull and forward into the light of Neon's eyes. As yet our two eyes cannot work in unison, hence there is no depth perception – the world appears flat and two-dimensional. Stereoscopic perception appears in Argon and with it the complexities of the third dimension. Conscious and subconscious minds mingle, throat chakras open and thyroid glands metabolize the elements of our bodies into living healthy organisms.

In the parallel biblical account the creation of Helios sun and light in Day One turns into the water project of Day Two, at the end of which Neon exposes the land, a flat firm base to stand on. In Day Three water and earth are separated, but will be reunited by the water cycle: Sun shines, clouds rise, wind blows, rain falls, seeds propagate and trees grow. Argon and its merry band of elements will render the earth fertile and burst into a three dimensional, self-sustaining world, a most beautiful garden to play in.

Every noble gas provides the answer to a question posed by the preceding period, while at the same time presenting a question to the following period. Neon poses the question of duality and Argon's response is to reunite Neon's division into a new oneness, marrying earth and water, land and sky, male and female into a three dimensional stereophonic choir of growth, childhood and joy. But while we yearn to conserve the timeless, naïve and carefree life of a child, preservation cannot last forever. This is the school of life, and we must forge forward seeking new problems and new solutions. Argon's question to the next period is: 'Excuse me, what is (the) time?'

The periodic table of our evolution is a one-way street. The gateway to childhood's garden closes behind us, guarded by the Tree of Logic. We must march to the beat of time, the journey to entropy. And so we are doomed to travel down the fourth period seeking temporal accommodation. There is but one way to reverse the process, to return to the source, and that is by finding the Tree of Life. This tree can only be discovered by internalising its essence. We must dive into its mirror.

This evolution can be summed up by the following synthesis:

Pre Creation (Nononium[i]): I am truly One.

Hydrogen: I have lost my oneness.

Helium's solution and problem: Delusion I am one, a line.

Neon's solution to Helium: Divide, splitting line into width; creating a two-dimensional surface.

Neon's pathology: Split in two, surface tension.

Neon's question to the third period: How will you deal with my division?

Argon's solution: Seek a new dimension. Learn to relate, and then unite two into one. Connect earth and water to grow a vertical tree. Height creates space.

Argon's pathology: Trying to preserve perfection, flow obstructed.

Argon's question to the fourth period and Krypton: How can I move forward?

Krypton's answer: Take your time, baby.

Time to move on and we are nearing the half-way mark.

The number three kept coming up all through the proving, over and over and over again. I feel four is embryonic, but now three is beginning to become four. Three is complete; once it's four it's over.

I kept getting lost and not recognising where I was in the mists. Am I halfway through creation?

For as much as you attempt to preserve, you cannot stop time forever.

Feels like time is ticking away – I'm waiting for what?

---

[i] Element Zero, the noble gas before creation. A term suggested by J Sherr.

Krypton encrypted

Apple fall, Newton call
Eins-time moving on,
We're diving through the mirror now
And heading for Krypton

Keppler counting, Rabbi blessing
Moon and sun revolve
Six and thirty puzzles here
That you cannot re-solve

Chambers pumping, heart is beating
One, two, three and four
Dalai Lama, hieroglyphics,
Who could ask for more?

So superman or batman?
Joker or a riddle?
The period we visit next
Is lying in the middle.

We meet in Krypton. Don't turn around.

Appendix A

This diagram (Figure App. 1) is based on the four elements and the four points between the elements. The intermediate points are Air-Water, which is a static energy (cold and wet-ice); Water-Fire, which is expansive (wet and hot-steam); Fire-Earth, which is dynamic (hot and dry) and finally Earth-Air, which is contractive (dry and cold, metal). This is the standard four element configuration that is well known in some homoeopathic circles. Onto this I have superimposed the elements of the first three periods laid out in a spiral, as well as the process of evolution of the soul and pregnancy (blue italics). The correspondences are quite instructive. We will be comparing the circle of four elements to the evolution of the periodic table, soul incarnation and pregnancy.

Begin at the top of the diagram and move clockwise. Fire corresponds to the singularity and to the Big Bang – all souls are one. This is also the point of orgasm before conception. Soon after the big bang, hydrogen is formed (Rudolf Steiner suggested it be called pyrogen – the fire element). Once hydrogen forms there is a separation from God that marks the first stages of the formation of an individual soul. Four hydrogen nuclei, or soul gametes, fuse into an individual Helium soul at the point of maximum expansion (suns and stars form). This corresponds to the point of conception, after which the embryonic cells start multiplying, and to the first day of creation, let there be light.[1]

The full soul now splits into two halves or soul mates, which incarnate as two hydrogen ions that combine with oxygen to form the Water of Life, H_2O. Thus life is initially the combination of fire and air, father and mother, together creating water, which fills the uterus during pregnancy. This corresponds to the second day of creation, the Water Story.

Now carbon and nitrogen form, creating physical structure and barriers respectively, while aligning with the point of maximum static, the material body. This is the beginning of the firmament, which culminates in ozone.

Oxygen and ozone naturally appear at the Air point, oxygen on the white/life side and ozone on the black/death side. At the corresponding time, towards the end of pregnancy, the fetal lungs develop. Fluoride then follows, with the highest electronegativity and reactivity of the periodic table – the ability to attract all other elements – and thus represents maximum contraction. This is analogous to the contraction of the waters into one place in Day Three, as well as the breaking of water just before birth. The newborn neon finally touches the earth, the 'last' of the four elements to appear. Neon lies on the Water/Earth axis, corresponding to

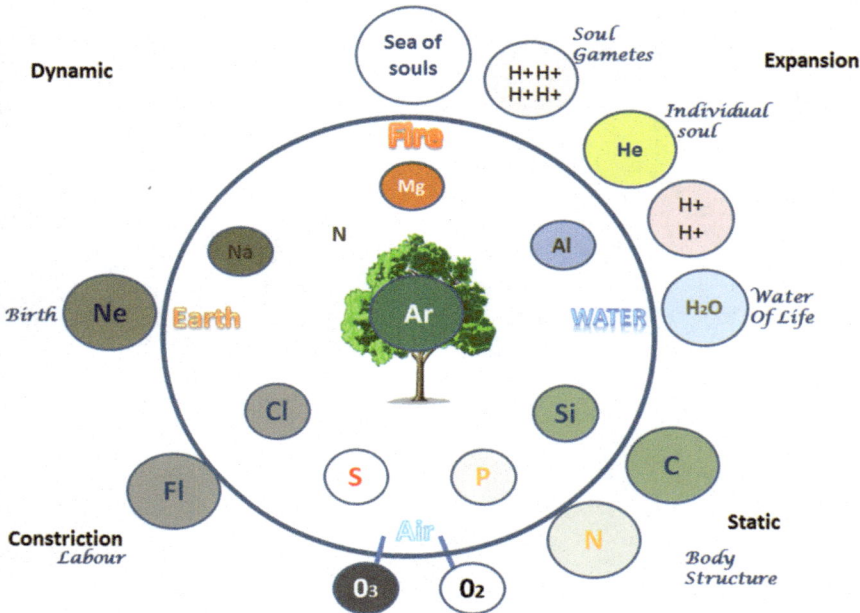

Figure App. 1 *Spiral periodic table.*

the biblical separation of earth and water. Between these two elements is the ozone firmament. (See Neon book for full explanation.)

The spiral now continues toward Argon. (At this point it would be useful to reexamine Camilla's meditation provings in Chapter 14.) Sodium corresponds to earth and salt and the brightly burning magnesium corresponds to fire. Alumina relates to expansion of identity, silica to static and structure, phosphorus to the consumptive oxygen, and sulphur to the misery of ozone, the dark firmament. The Chlorine proving is well known for its contractive powers. Finally, we spiral into the center, the perfect Tree of Life, Argon, a combination of Fire, Air, Water and Earth.

Reference

1.   Sherr J. *The Noble Gases. Helium including an introduction to the Noble Gases.* Glasgow: Saltire Books, 2011. p71.

INDEX

Note: (*fn*) refers to footnote.